FIRESIDE

"*Nutrition for the Working Woman* belongs in every kitchen, next to a favorite cookbook. It's chock-full of sound, practical information that will take the worry out of nutrition, cooking and meal planning."

—Kristen McNutt, Esq., Ph.D.
Associate Director of the
Good Housekeeping Institute

NUTRITION for the WORKING WOMAN

Audrey Tittle Cross, J.D., M.P.H.

A Fireside Book
Published by Simon & Schuster, Inc.
New York

The author is grateful for permission to reprint lyrics from "Big Boss Man" by
Al Smith and Luther Dixon, © 1960 and 1967 by Conrad Music, a Division
of Arc Music Corporation. All rights reserved.

Simon and Schuster/Fireside Books
Published by Simon & Schuster, Inc.
Simon & Schuster Building
Rockefeller Center
1230 Avenue of the Americas
New York, New York 10020
SIMON and SCHUSTER, FIRESIDE and colophons
are registered trademarks
of Simon & Schuster, Inc.

Designed by Jennie Nichols/Levavi & Levavi
Manufactured in the United States of America

10 9 8 7 6 5 4 3 2 1

Library of Congress Cataloging in Publication Data
Cross, Audrey Tittle.
  Nutrition for the working woman.

  "A Fireside book."
  Bibliography: p.
  Includes index.
  1. Nutrition. 2. Women—Employment. 3. Women—Time manage-
ment. 4. Home economics. 5. Family—Health and hygiene. I. Title.
RA784.C68 1985 613.2'024042 85-12950
ISBN: 0-671-61707-9
ISBN: 0-671-54069-6 Pbk.

Acknowledgments

I never really dreamed about writing a book. It seemed like too long and lonely a task, and a risky one, since there was no guarantee that anyone other than my mother would love it!

Dr. Mark Hegsted, now at the Primate Research Facility at Harvard Medical School, first prodded me, saying, "Why not? Everyone else has written a nutrition book." Dr. Elizabeth Sloane, director of the Good Housekeeping Institute, introduced me to my agent, Perry Belmont Frank. With his partner, Norman Monath, a publisher was secured. To each of them, for their encouragement and assistance, I am grateful.

I am particularly grateful to Barbara Gess, my editor, for her kindness and understanding during my mother's death while I was writing this book. Barbara graciously allowed me the time that I needed to spend the last months of Mother's life with her.

The help of the Sociology Department at Stanford University is also appreciated. During Mother's hospitalization at Stanford Medical Center, the department gave me free use of a computer to continue work on the book during the evenings.

A very special thanks to the nutritional sciences faculty of the University of California, Berkeley, especially Drs. Doris Calloway and Sheldon Margen, by whom I was trained. Their commitment to the study and teaching of the science and art of nutrition is a continuing source of direction and inspiration for me.

And finally, my thanks to my husband, who cheered me on when I felt overcome by circumstances. He fervently believes that women have a nearly limitless ability as managers. He expresses his continual amazement that we can pursue a career *and* run a household, since he knows few men who could do both with any degree of finesse. He very much wanted me to share with you the things I do to make this double task easy, effortless, and satisfying.

To my mother, whose untimely death from cancer during the writing of this book robbed her of the joy of seeing it in print.

To my father, Fred C. Tittle, who is a constant source of love, inspiration, and funny stories.

To my 85-year-old grandmother, Lillian Hibdon, who taught me much that I know about managing family and food.

To my husband, Steven Gambino, who stands behind me when I advocate that we women seize the helm of the household and run it like General Motors.

And to my stepdaughter, Jennifer, who is only just beginning to know her full power and potential as a woman.

Contents

INTRODUCTION   13

1. BALANCING IT ALL—THE ESTABLISHMENT OF
   HOME, INC.   15
   Getting Started   19

2. YOUR MANAGEMENT OBJECTIVES   21
   Nutritional Objectives   22
   Individual Components: The Nutrients   28
   Supplements   71
   Production Component Summary   79

3. TRIMMING THE FAT   80
   Standards of Weights and Measures   81
   Fit or Fat?   83
   Fat and Forty   87
   Mirror, Mirror   88
   Is a Calorie Always a Calorie?   91

4. HOME, INC., BUSINESS PLAN   100
   Menus to End Muddling Through   101
   How It Works   103
   Putting It into Patterns   110
   Vegetarians   113
   Pregnancy and Lactation   118
   Infant Feeding   121
   Planning Family Menus   123
   Seven Days of Menus   125

5. CONTINGENCY PLANS   129
   Snacking   129
   Bagging It   132
   Dieting Out   137
   "It Cannot Work for Me Because My Life Does Not
      Look Like That!"   141
   The Final Frontier   144
   Cooking It Right   148

6. PURCHASING SUPPLIES FOR HOME, INC.   154
   Do Dollars Stretch?   155
   Fuss Budget   155
   Inventory Management   157
   Locating Suppliers   159
   Better Buys for the Buck   162
   Fruit and Vegetable Groups   164
   Dairy Foods Group   176
   Carbohydrate Foods Group   181
   Protein Foods Group   187
   Processed, Packaged, Fluffed, and Puffed   196
   Nutritionally Economic Foods—The Very Best Buys   203

7. MANAGEMENT MANEUVERS—SAVING TIME
   AND MONEY   205
   Time Is Money   205
   Cutting Shopping Time   207
   Equipment   210
   Doing Ahead   223

Timing Meal Preparation   225
Cleanup   229

8. RECYCLING AND REFUSE—LEFTOVERS   234
Recycling   236
Storage   239

9. MARKETING YOUR PRODUCT   241
Setting a Pretty Table   242
Places to Eat   243
Coverings   243
Centerpieces   245
Lighting   245
Food Presentation   246
What You Call It   249

10. MARKET TRENDS   251
Fashionable Foods   253
Spotting Trends   255
Riding the Shirttails of Trend Setters   255
Succeeding   257

APPENDIX   259
Management Work Sheets   259
Food Groups   263
Checklist   266
Shopping List   266
Delegation   267

INDEX   271

Introduction

As an active and busy woman, I often dream of having a "wife"
—that wonderfully warm, cheerful, and loving soul who would
greet me at the door with a drink, a few hors d'oeuvres to hold
my appetite until dinnertime and ears sympathetic to the woes
of my day.

Never again would I want for my morning coffee. It would be
ready when I walked out of the shower. My dieter's brown-bag
lunch would be waiting patiently at the front door to accompany
me to the office. Before the knock of the first guest, flowers
would be arranged, the table would be simply but elegantly set,
and dinner would be ready to pop into the oven.

The family food and beverages budget would be managed as
efficiently as a four-star restaurant. Groceries and household supplies would appear on schedule like a Southern Pacific locomo-
tive. Nutritional needs of each family member would be
balanced with Mayo Clinic precision, and we would be healthy,
trim, and athletic, appetite appeased and pleased!

As fortune would have it, like you, I get to *be* the wife rather
than to have one! Yet I do believe in having my dreams instead
of just dreaming them. So I have devised some fairy godmother-
like schemes which help me to balance my budget, bulges, and
binges.

It is not impossible! What is required is a bit less time frantically fighting crisis in the kitchen and more time thinking, planning, and delegating. I have seized control of my kitchen and now run it like a small corporation of which I am chief executive officer.

No more wringing my hands and wondering what to cook for dinner. No more worrying about whether everyone is getting the nutrients they need. No more disappointment that my dinner parties leave out too many details to qualify as really elegant. No more time "alligators" swallowing up my evenings. No more waste of precious food dollars.

Borrowing techniques from managers in the business world, I have devised a plan to:

○ Meet the nutritional requirements of all family members
○ Keep calories in check
○ Serve elegant and appetizing meals
○ Expend a minimum amount of time and energy
○ Use natural and fresh ingredients
○ While living within a budget

I offer it to you here.

1. Balancing It All—the Establishment of Home, Inc.

Whether we work outside our homes or not, whether we are deeply involved in community and civic activities or not, whether we have household help or not, we still run the kitchen. Whether we like it or not, women are ultimately the people in charge of managing and operating the kitchen.

To be successful at a job, we must first admit that it *is* our job. The job really does not belong to our husbands, though they certainly may help out to lesser or greater degrees. The job does not belong to our children, though they too may pitch in to help. But when there is a question about what to do next, or a catastrophe or problem to solve, you are the one they ask for a decision. Because you are in charge!

Many of us like to pretend that the job will do itself; that delicious and well-balanced meals will happen without guidance or supervision. There are some laws of nature like that: what goes up does come down; water does run downhill. But kitchens do not run themselves. A kitchen with no one in charge produces haphazard meals which randomly meet individual family member nutrition needs and swallow a larger share of family fortune than is necessary. A job simply does not get done if no one is in charge.

You may have hundreds of good reasons why you do not want to be the one in charge. They range from "I hate to cook" to

"I don't have time" to "It is not socially important work" to "It does not pay well" to "I'd rather be sailing." Unfortunately, none of those answers changes the fact that you are in charge.

"But I hate to cook!"

Whether you love it or hate it, you are still responsible for what gets cooked. You can delegate the actual doing of the cooking to a family member, maid, or to convenience foods manufacturers. But you are still in charge of the total job, and cooking is only one part of it.

"I don't have time!"

Chances are you also think that you do not have time for a whole list of other things in life. What is needed is not more time, but more time management. Management is the responsibility of the person in charge. You are in charge.

"It's not socially significant work."

The job is not only central to the family's social well-being, it is also crucial to their health. When the job is not done, the family suffers in spirit and in body. And as a functioning economic unit, the family suffers financially when the kitchen is not managed. The job is socially significant, financially critical, and medically important.

"It doesn't pay well."

A poorly done job never pays well. A poorly managed kitchen squanders hundreds of dollars annually in low-nutrient food choices, in overpriced purchases, and in food waste. By contrast, a well-managed kitchen provides delicious meals which meet family nutrient needs, are fun and appetizing, time-efficient, waste-sparing, and dollar-saving.

"I'd rather be sailing!"

A managed kitchen does not consume excessive amounts of your time. A managed kitchen runs like a tight ship with all hands on deck. It can provide you with the health, energy, and leftover money to go sailing!

So! It is time to tell the truth. You are the person in charge. You are responsible. You are THE person whose decisions make or break your family's nutritional health and the health of a major portion of the family budget.

I have lectured and spoken to thousands of you across the nation. And one theme is clear. You want to run your home with the same level of efficiency, expertise, warmth, and devotion as you would if you had the luxury to devote your full time and attention to the job. All those reasons and excuses about why you "can't" or "don't" are the voices of your own fears and disappointments about not doing the job as well as you would like.

For many of you achieving that dream may seem overwhelming and unmanageable. There may seem to be just too many small details, too many decisions to make about nutrients and food sources of nutrients, and costs, and scheduling and preparation and presentation. This "can't-see-the-forest-for-the-trees" syndrome may lead you to daydream, "If only things were different."

The difference between dreams and reality is action. A dream which is not acted upon has no more value than the vapor rising from your morning coffee as you dream it.

Achieving dreams is a matter of taking control and acting. It is a matter of recognizing that you are the source of having your dreams come true. You are your own fairy godmother. Your kitchen will run like clockwork when you organize it and order it to do so. Left to itself, your kitchen will erode into chaos and confusion.

Henry Ford did not build an automobile manufacturing plant and expect it to produce cars by itself. You cannot own a kitchen and expect it to produce meals without you. Mr. Ford first appointed himself the one in charge. He declared that he was the boss, the manager, the chairman of the board, the chief executive officer.

Then he did what chief executive officers do. He defined what his product was and what it would do. He made a list of what components he needed to make it. He decided where he would purchase the needed components. He calculated how much money he would need to finance his project—both for goods to be used in products and for the equipment to do the production. He studied how to keep costs and waste down. He examined ways to market or advertise his product to sell it. And he set up a system to monitor continually how well his product was being received by his customers.

Henry Ford had a plan. The difference between a dream and a plan is action.

The chapters which follow are designed to assist you in taking control of your own small business, Home, Inc. First, I invite you to seize the helm. Take responsibility (and take credit!) for the job which you are already doing. You are the boss, so give yourself a title. Call yourself the boss.

In case you are shy about making lofty pronouncements, maybe this will help you out: I hereby appoint you chief executive officer of your own Home, Inc. (How does that feel? Maybe you should have business cards made up!)

What follows is a manual for managing your own Home, Inc. It is formulas for balancing your budget, bulges, and binges. It is a road map to success.

In your new position as CEO, your first task will be to define corporate purpose and goals. Mine are to achieve:

1. Optimal health and well-being for each family member
2. At a normal body weight
3. While living within a food budget
4. And presenting food that is delicious, easy, entertaining, and attractive

To begin, you will need information on what nutrients are needed and in what amounts to achieve optimal health. Chapter 2 will brief you on criteria for setting these goals. It will examine recommended levels of nutrient intake and what the importance of each nutrient is. This is similar to Henry Ford learning that automobiles are sturdier when constructed from steel than from straw.

Chapter 3 will assist you in defining the limits of girth for family members: who is fat, who is fit, what is fattening, and how to turn it around. Mr. Ford could not build a battleship-size car with a Model T–size motor. The burdensome size would wear out the motor.

You will next need to chart your plan of action. The chapters which follow tell you "how to" get it done. Now that you know that everybody needs calcium, how do you buy it and cook it? How do you know whether you are stocking too much of the wrong thing from the wrong supplier?

Like Mr. Ford's action plans, these chapters detail:

○ How to write input specifications (menus)
○ How to order and inventory component supplies (shopping and staples lists)
○ Supplies purchasing and acquisition techniques (how to buy it better, cheaper)
○ Assembling skills (cooking it right)

Once you get the menus written, the food stocked, and assembling skills mastered, you are ready to "hire staff." Under training and supervision of assembly-line personnel, you will learn how to turn one husband, the kids, and a microwave into Sara Lee Kitchens!

Like Henry Ford, you will find that at the end of each operating cycle you have "spare parts"—unused or leftover pieces and portions. Should you call your church soup kitchen to donate them or feed them to your dog or garbage disposal? You will learn how every good manager from Henry Ford to Lee Iacocca recycles leftovers.

Were it not for advertisement, few of us would know the difference between Revlon and Pond's face creams. They look the same in the jar and serve the same purpose. You will learn how to "package" and "promote" your meals to turn bean stew into cassoulet.

Finally, you will learn how to track trends in order to keep family meals in pace with changing food preferences. Two years ago all they would eat was chicken. Now you have three frozen chickens drying out in the freezer because this year everyone wants to eat veal with the president. Henry Ford II got stuck with only a dozen or so Edsels in the warehouse because he stopped production when he saw demand fall off.

If you are wondering if there are forms which you can buy at the office supply store which will make this whole job easier, there are not. There are no yellow pads that you rub with a pencil to reveal invisible answers. But there are work sheets in the back of this book which you can copy and reuse for planning, stocking supplies, and scheduling work.

GETTING STARTED

You may at first fumble with the details of managing family nutrition. Writing menus may seem difficult. Organizing a shopping list may seem to take more time than it is worth. Saving a few pennies here or there may seem too tedious. Changing table decor may seem unnecessary.

Quality is produced by attention to detail and skill. Skill results from repetition. Fine crafts people are relentless in their training, repeating and repeating each move until it is perfect and every detail is right. Ultimately excellence becomes automatic and their craft is no longer difficult. It looks easy and is easy.

Excellence is a commitment. It is a desire to turn the impersonal into the personal. It is that extra thought and caring which distinguishes it from the mundane. It is the out of the ordinary. Excellence is a distinction.

It is a habit. As a habit, excellence is just as easy as any other. You can habitually serve the same old tired meals or you can get into the habit of varying your menus. You can habitually eat at the same table setting, or you can get into the habit of varying where and how meals are served.

As you strive for excellence in the practice of your new role as CEO, notice the effect that you produce on your family. Notice how easy and effortless getting meals to the table becomes when you have a system and delegate tasks to helpers. Notice the extra dollars that begin to accumulate in the food budget. Notice the response of guests and family to the ambiance of your food and table presentations. Notice how much less hassled you feel about food and nutrition when the kitchen is in control. And notice, how, after a while, it all seems effortless and automatic.

Let's get started.

2. Your Management Objectives

An almost unlimited variety of foods are available to us—everything from imported Russian caviar to domestic aged cheese to imported Australian lamb and domestic wild rice. And whether it is winter or summer, Maine or Michigan, ripe California avocados and tomatoes await our purchase. It would seem easy to be well nourished.

Surprisingly, we don't always do the best job of selecting foods. The federal government regularly collects information on American eating patterns and on the health impact of these choices. It reports that we are not doing as well as we could. Our habits are getting even worse.

Every ten years the U.S. Department of Agriculture conducts a survey of foods families eat. Over the years, significant changes have occurred in what we commonly eat. For example, in 1910 about 32 percent of the calories in our diets came from fat. By 1976 we consumed more than 42 percent of our calories as fat. Our intake of soft drinks had increased by 157 percent, while our intake of fresh fruit had decreased by 33 percent.

A Health and Nutrition Examination Survey (HANES) is conducted approximately every three years by the federal government to determine the health consequences of these changes in our eating patterns. Diseases and health problems resulting from too little food, such as goiter, beriberi, and scurvy, are rarely found in the United States. However, the survey has uncovered an increasing number of health problems related to excesses in the diet, such as obesity, heart disease, and diabetes.

Eating is a necessity. But what we eat is a matter of habit. Just as selection of low-quality input components produces poor products in the manufacturing industries, so can poor eating habits contribute to poor health and fitness.

NUTRITIONAL OBJECTIVES

Lee Iacocca oversees a multimillion-dollar business concerned with the essential components and parts to build automobiles. His objective is to produce a car which functions properly, is stylish, requires minimum upkeep and maintenance, and is available at an affordable price.

As CEO in charge of Home, Inc., we face decisions equal in importance to those of the president of Chrysler Motor Company. While we do not formally state them, families have purposes, goals, and objectives just like corporations do. And just like corporations, certain components are required. How wisely we select those components, their cost-benefit ratio, will determine how well we meet the family's health and fitness goals.

The building materials or manufacturing components with which we work are chemical substances called nutrients. Over 45 in total are required for our bodies to grow, move, think, and make repairs.

When Mr. Iacocca's company needs carburetors, he must determine the construction materials, design specifications, performance standards, and cost criteria which his suppliers must meet before he will buy their carburetors. When choosing between food sources of a nutrient, you will also need some guidelines and specifications. How much is enough, too little, or too much? Is one nutrient more important than another? Is every form in which the nutrient occurs equally usable for the purpose? Is a less expensive form just as efficient and effective as a more expensive form? Can costs be safely cut on some nutrients but not on others?

Let's look at our "manufacturing components" to see what criteria might best guide our food choices.

Critical Criteria for Components

When we ingest food, our bodies break it down during digestion into its chemical constituents, called nutrients. These nutrients are absorbed and then used by the body to build and repair its parts or to operate its many functions. This process is called metabolism.

Every minute of the day, whether we are sleeping or playing racquetball, our bodies are involved in this process. The basic functioning of our bodies—beating of the heart, activity of the brain, breathing, muscle tone, etc.—is called basal metabolism. Together our basal metabolism and physical activity (walking, writing) make up our total need for energy.

Only three components of food—protein, carbohydrate, and fat—supply energy, which we measure in calories. Vitamins and minerals help our bodies to release and use the energy from these nutrients. They do not provide calories. Additionally, vitamins and minerals have specific functions which only they can perform.

Our bodies cannot manufacture their own supply of vitamins or minerals. It is essential that we get them from our food supply. Only small amounts are needed daily; however, a shortage can lead to specific deficiency diseases, like rickets and pellagra.

Fortunately, you will not have to hire a team of designers, engineers, draftsmen, and so forth to figure how much of each of these nutrients you and your family members need. "Specifications" already exist. The National Academy of Sciences/National Research Council's Food and Nutrition Board, a group of nationally eminent nutrition researchers and scientists, meets every three to five years to establish these "specifications," called the "Recommended Dietary Allowances" or "RDA" (see Table 2.1, Recommended Daily Dietary Allowances, and Table 2.2, estimates for nutrients for which no RDAs have been established).

Notice that these are only recommendations. The RDAs are estimates of the amount of essential nutrients which will meet the needs of the majority of healthy persons in the United States. They are based on studies of groups of people. Therefore they do not really apply to the specific nutrient needs of individuals. In fact, they are set slightly higher than what any one individual may require to ensure a margin of safety.

TABLE 2.1 FOOD AND NUTRITION BOARD, NATIONAL ACADEMY OF SCIENCES—NATIONAL RESEARCH COUNCIL RECOMMENDED DAILY DIETARY ALLOWANCES,[a] Revised 1980

(Designed for the maintenance of good nutrition of practically all healthy people in the U.S.A.)

Age (years)	Weight (kg)	Weight (lb)	Height (cm)	Height (in.)	Protein (g)	Fat-Soluble Vitamins			Water-Soluble Vitamins							Minerals					
						Vitamin A (μg RE)[b]	Vitamin D (μg)[c]	Vitamin E (mg α-TE)[d]	Vitamin C (mg)	Thiamin (mg)	Riboflavin (mg)	Niacin (mg NE)[e]	Vitamin B-6 (mg)	Folacin (μg)[f]	Vitamin B-12 (μg)	Calcium (mg)	Phosphorus (mg)	Magnesium (mg)	Iron (mg)	Zinc (mg)	Iodine (μg)
Infants																					
0.0-0.5	6	13	60	24	kg × 2.2	420	10	3	35	0.3	0.4	6	0.3	30	0.5[g]	360	240	50	10	3	40
0.5-1.0	9	20	71	28	kg × 2.0	400	10	4	35	0.5	0.6	8	0.6	45	1.5	540	360	70	15	5	50
Children																					
1-3	13	29	90	35	23	400	10	5	45	0.7	0.8	9	0.9	100	2.0	800	800	150	15	10	70
4-6	20	44	112	44	30	500	10	6	45	0.9	1.0	11	1.3	200	2.5	800	800	200	10	10	90
7-10	28	62	132	52	34	700	10	7	45	1.2	1.4	16	1.6	300	3.0	800	800	250	10	10	120
Males																					
11-14	45	99	157	62	45	1000	10	8	50	1.4	1.6	18	1.8	400	3.0	1200	1200	350	18	15	150
15-18	66	145	176	69	56	1000	10	10	60	1.4	1.7	18	2.0	400	3.0	1200	1200	400	18	15	150
19-22	70	154	177	70	56	1000	7.5	10	60	1.5	1.7	19	2.2	400	3.0	800	800	350	10	15	150
23-50	70	154	178	70	56	1000	5	10	60	1.4	1.6	18	2.2	400	3.0	800	800	350	10	15	150
51+	70	154	178	70	56	1000	5	10	60	1.2	1.4	16	2.2	400	3.0	800	800	350	10	15	150
Females																					
11-14	46	101	157	62	46	800	10	8	50	1.1	1.3	15	1.8	400	3.0	1200	1200	300	18	15	150
15-18	55	120	163	64	46	800	10	8	60	1.1	1.3	14	2.0	400	3.0	1200	1200	300	18	15	150
19-22	55	120	163	64	44	800	7.5	8	60	1.1	1.3	14	2.0	400	3.0	800	800	300	18	15	150
23-50	55	120	163	64	44	800	5	8	60	1.0	1.2	13	2.0	400	3.0	800	800	300	18	15	150
51+	55	120	163	64	44	800	5	8	60	1.0	1.2	13	2.0	400	3.0	800	800	300	10	15	150
Pregnant					+30	+200	+5	+2	+20	+0.4	+0.3	+2	+0.6	+400	+1.0	+400	+400	+150	h	+5	+25
Lactating					+20	+400	+5	+3	+40	+0.5	+0.5	+5	+0.5	+100	+1.0	+400	+400	+150	h	+10	+50

[a] The allowances are intended to provide for individual variations among most normal persons as they live in the United States under usual environmental stresses. Diets should be based on a variety of common foods in order to provide other nutrients for which human requirements have been less well defined.

[b] Retinol equivalents: 1 retinol equivalent = 1 μg retinol or 6 μg β carotene.

[c] As cholecalciferol, 10 μg cholecalciferol = 400 IU of vitamin D.

[d] α-tocopherol equivalents. 1 mg d-α tocopherol = 1 α-TE. See text for variation in allowances and calculation of vitamin E activity of the diet as α-tocopherol equivalents.

[e] 1 NE (niacin equivalent) is equal to 1 mg of niacin or 60 mg of dietary tryptophan.

[f] The folacin allowances refer to dietary sources as determined by Lactobacillus casei assay after treatment with enzymes (conjugases) to make polyglutamyl forms of the vitamin available to the test organism.

[g] The recommended dietary allowances for vitamin B-12 in infants is based on average concentration of the vitamin in human milk. The allowances after weaning are based on energy intake (as recommended by the American Academy of Pediatrics) and consideration of other factors, such as intestinal absorption.

[h] The increased requirement during pregnancy cannot be met by the iron content of habitual American diets nor by the existing iron stores of many women; therefore the use of 30–60 mg of supplemental iron is recommended. Iron needs during lactation are not substantially different from those of nonpregnant women, but continued supplementation of the mother for 2–3 months after parturition is advisable in order to replenish stores depleted by pregnancy.

Source: Adapted from "Recommended Dietary Allowances," 9th revised edition, 1980, with permission of the National Academy Press, Washington, D.C.

TABLE 2.2 ESTIMATED SAFE AND ADEQUATE DAILY DIETARY INTAKES OF SELECTED VITAMINS AND MINERALS[a]

Vitamins

	Age (years)	Vitamin K (μg)	Biotin (μg)	Panto-thenic Acid (mg)
Infants	0–0.5	12	35	2
	0.5–1	10–20	50	3
Children	1–3	15–30	65	3
and	4–6	20–40	85	3–4
Adolescents	7–10	30–60	120	4–5
	11+	50–100	100–200	4–7
Adults		70–140	100–200	4–7

Trace Elements[b]

	Age (years)	Copper (mg)	Man-ganese (mg)	Fluoride (mg)	Chromium (mg)	Selenium (mg)	Molyb-denum (mg)
Infants	0–0.5	0.5–0.7	0.5–0.7	0.1–0.5	0.01–0.04	0.01–0.04	0.03–0.06
	0.5–1	0.7–1.0	0.7–1.0	0.2–1.0	0.02–0.06	0.02–0.06	0.04–0.08
Children	1–3	1.0–1.5	1.0–1.5	0.5–1.5	0.02–0.08	0.02–0.08	0.05–0.1
and	4–6	1.5–2.0	1.5–2.0	1.0–2.5	0.03–0.12	0.03–0.12	0.06–0.15
Adolescents	7–10	2.0–2.5	2.0–3.0	1.5–2.5	0.05–0.2	0.05–0.2	0.10–0.3
	11+	2.0–3.0	2.5–5.0	1.5–2.5	0.05–0.2	0.05–0.2	0.15–0.5
Adults		2.0–3.0	2.5–5.0	1.5–4.0	0.05–0.2	0.05–0.2	0.15–0.5

Electrolytes

	Age (years)	Sodium (mg)	Potassium (mg)	Chloride (mg)
Infants	0–0.5	115–350	350–925	275–700
	0.5–1	250–750	425–1275	400–1200
Children	1–3	325–975	550–1650	500–1500
and	4–6	450–1350	775–2325	700–2100
Adolescents	7–10	600–1800	1000–3000	925–2775
	11+	900–2700	1525–4575	1400–4200
Adults		1100–3300	1875–5625	1700–5100

[a] Because there is less information on which to base allowances, these figures are not given in the main table of RDA and are provided here in the form of ranges of recommended intakes.

[b] Since the toxic levels for many trace elements may be only several times usual intakes, the upper levels for the trace elements given in this table should not be habitually exceeded.

Source: Reproduced from "Recommended Dietary Allowances," 1980.

Even with these limitations, the RDAs are still good guide-posts to follow.

Labels on Components

The RDAs are not to be confused with the USRDA which you commonly see on cereal boxes, food labels, and vitamin/mineral supplements. The USRDA was devised by the Food and Drug Administration (FDA) in an effort to give consumers information about the nutrients in their foods.

Foods are analyzed to see how much of each nutrient is in a serving. By itself, this value is not very useful. You also need to know how much of the nutrient you need each day. So the amount of nutrient in the serving is expressed as a percentage of the amount you need. It tells you whether one serving contains 100 percent or 60 percent of the vitamin C you need.

You notice on the RDA chart that each nutrient has a standard for each age and sex. As you can imagine, it would be impossible to print the percentage of even one nutrient for each of these groups on the wrapper of a Snickers candy bar!

Therefore the FDA decided to use a single standard for each nutrient, the USRDA. This standard is based on the RDA but is not age/sex specific. So there is only one value for each nutrient. Generally the USRDA is the highest recommended intake level for any nutrient. For example, the highest RDA for vitamin A is 5000 IU (international units) so this is the value used for the USRDA.

Clearly it would also be impractical to require that information on all the nutrients in a food be listed. Therefore, the FDA requires that manufacturers list information only for those nutrients about which they have made an advertising claim or any nutrients which they have added. For example, if an advertisement states "high in protein" or "low in cholesterol," then it must have a nutrient label with specific facts to substantiate this claim.

If a manufacturer makes no advertising claims and adds no nutrients, then it is not required to put nutrient information on the label. If a manufacturer does decide to label a food voluntarily, then it must list calories per serving, protein, carbohydrate, and fat content in grams per serving; and the percentage USRDA from protein, vitamins A and C, thiamine, riboflavin, niacin, calcium, and iron.

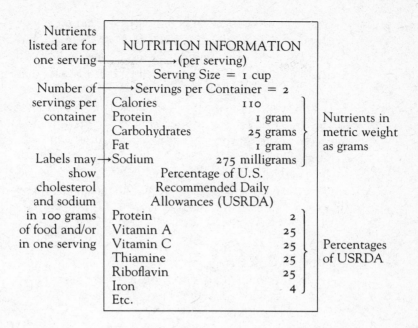

How nutrient information appears on a label is shown in the chart. Notice that all nutritional information is listed in terms of single servings. A single serving is a standard measurement and may not reflect the actual portion consumed. For example, frozen vegetables come in 10-ounce boxes which are designated as serving four. We find them to contain barely enough for three. Therefore the nutrient values per serving do not apply to our family because we eat larger portions of vegetables than the container specifies for "one serving."

As troublesome as it may seem, the benefit of reading labels is to judge product quality better. Food labels are designed to help consumers understand nutrient density, that is, the number or relative amount of vitamins and minerals supplied by a food. It allows you to compare the number of nutrients available per calorie or per cost.

Other Operating Instructions

The RDA and USRDA focus on getting enough of those nutrients which we know to be essential to good health. In the past, diseases from lack of sufficient intakes of vitamins and minerals were common. In the late 1970s nutritionists began to worry about the opposite problem: excessive intakes of nutrients.

You cannot put too much oil in the crankcase of your car without problems, nor too much food in the body without consequences. Research findings point increasingly to the role of particular food and diet excesses in heart disease, obesity, cancer, and diabetes.

Today these diseases are far more common than deficiency diseases. Nutritionists decided that it was time to make recommendations about the hazards of too much as well as those of too little food.

In 1979, the U.S. Departments of Agriculture and Health and Human Services issued seven dietary guidelines to reduce the risk of these major diseases.

1. Eat a variety of foods.
2. Maintain ideal weight.
3. Avoid too much fat, saturated fat, and cholesterol.
4. Eat foods with adequate starch and fiber.
5. Avoid too much sugar.
6. Avoid too much sodium.
7. If you drink alcohol, do so in moderation.

The first guideline does reemphasize the importance of eating a wide variety of foods in order to ensure an adequate intake of the essential nutrients which our bodies need. The second guideline warns us not to exceed our ideal body weight, emphasizing the relationship between obesity, overweight, and the risk of diseases like cancer, heart and kidney disease, and strokes. Guidelines 3, 4, and 5 deal with the very habits which can lead to weight gain. Guidelines 6 and 7 are directed at those who abuse salt and alcohol, pointing out the associated health risks.

The American Heart Association with an endorsement by the American Medical Association, the National Cancer Institute, and the American Cancer Society have all released very similar suggestions for dietary changes to reduce the risk of chronic and killer diseases.

INDIVIDUAL COMPONENTS: THE NUTRIENTS

Now a bit more detailed information about each of the nutrients, their role in our health, and the consequences of extremely low or high intakes. Table 2.13 on pages 74–78 lists the role of each of the nutrients, food sources, deficiency symptoms, and effects of overdoses.

The discussion below will give you recent information on controversies, myths, and rumors about nutrients which you might have heard.

Carbohydrates

Until a few years ago, when we heard the word "carbohydrate" we saw chubby cherubs eating bonbons and bloating bigger and bigger. Or we pictured a stout Italian Mama with an apron the size of a tablecloth, cheerfully offering more pasta. "Carbohydrate" was a fattening word.

In truth, carbohydrates are, the world over, the major source of energy for the body. They are the staple food of mankind. And, as we will see, they are not fattening, per se.

There are several types of carbohydrates. All of them are made of the chemicals carbon (C), hydrogen (H), and oxygen (O) strung together in chains of varying length. The short chains, called "simple" carbohydrates, are sugars which are found in milk and fruit and in table sugars and in other sweeteners manufactured from beets, cane, corn, and other plants.

$$\underset{H}{\overset{O}{\diagup}}C - \underset{OH}{\overset{H}{C}} - \underset{OH}{\overset{H}{C}} - \underset{OH}{\overset{H}{C}} - \underset{OH}{\overset{H}{C}} - \underset{OH}{\overset{H}{C}} - OH \quad \text{is the sugar, glucose}$$

The long chains, called "complex" carbohydrates, are either starches or cellulose. Starches are found in grains and starchy vegetables like potatoes. Cellulose is not digestible so it provides no energy but it does provide fiber which we call bulk or roughage (see page 37).

Simple Sweets

Simple carbohydrates are the body's major source of fuel or energy. They include table sugar, honey, corn syrup, grape sugar, corn and other sweeteners, sorghum, maple, the sugars which occur in milk, fruits, and vegetables.

We are a nation of sugarholics and often consume far more sugars than we need for energy. According to U.S. Department of Agriculture studies, we consume, on the average, over 138

pounds apiece each year (1978). At that rate, we are not just
eating sugar by the teaspoon on our breakfast cereal! We are
eating more like 14 tablespoons a day, more than 600 calories
from sugars and sweeteners. Between 13–16 percent of the calories in the diet of children aged 1 to 18 and from 9 to 13 percent
of the calories consumed by adults are from sugar and refined
sweeteners.

We drink the majority of this sugar in soft drinks—21 percent. Another 18 percent is consumed as syrups, jellies, jams,
gelatin desserts, ices, Popsicles, and table sugar. Bakery products, including cakes, cookies, pies, pastries, and sweet crackers,
provide 13 percent of our sugar intake. The rest comes from
other snack foods, ice cream, sherbet, fruits packed in heavy
syrup, sugar-coated breakfast cereals, and hidden in prepared
entrées, canned and frozen vegetables, soups, mayonnaise, peanut butter, flavored yogurt, and just about every manufactured
food.

You will have to read food labels to know whether sugar has
been added. Often the chemical names of sugar are used to
disguise their presence. Following are some examples. Remember that these sugars are created equal! A sugar is a sugar is a
sugar, even when it assumes a fancy-sounding name as listed
here:

Brown sugar	Honey
Corn sweeteners	Lactose
Corn syrup	Maltose
Dextrin	Maple syrup
Dextrose	Molasses
Fructose	Raw sugar
Glucose	Turbinado

By law, ingredients are listed "in order of preponderance" on the
label. So if your breakfast cereal lists "sugar" as the first ingredient, you can bet that there is more sugar there than snap,
crackle, or pop.

Changes in FDA laws in 1984 may give the impression that
less sugar was added to a product than in fact was. Manufacturers
are now allowed to group similar food ingredients such as flours.
So, a breakfast cereal which actually contains more sugar than
either wheat and corn flours, might now read, "Wheat and corn
flours, sugar, etc." Since the grains can be grouped, it appears

that there is less sugar than flour. If the flours could not be grouped, the label would read, "Sugar, wheat flour, corn flour . . ."

Abusive intake of sugars can contribute to weight gain. Those 500–600 extra calories which we consume daily as sugar can add up to a gradual gain of 10 pounds in a year. Since much of the sugar we eat is hidden in our foods, we might be mystified as to the source of those excess calories. As our weight edges upward, so does the risk of diabetes and heart disease. Sugar doesn't cause these diseases directly. But it clearly is the culprit in a great deal of the girth of America!

SWEET TOOTH

Tooth decay is another sugar risk. Sticky, gooey sweet foods which adhere to the tooth surface provide a great growing ground for the bacteria which cause tooth decay. Americans spend billions of dollars each year on dental bills. By the time the average American child is 16, he or she has at least 11 missing, filled, or decayed teeth. If you are not going to moderate your family's intakes of sugar then you should at least rush out to purchase more toothbrushes and a dental insurance policy.

SUGAR SLUMP

Simple sugars are also implicated in "midmorning Blahs," that tired, listless feeling that hits just before lunchtime. The Blahs are common to people who grab a sugar-glazed doughnut and coffee with sugar and cream as they hit the highway, bound onto the bus, stumble into the subway, or dash to their desk just before the clock strikes.

The body has fasted through the night. Instead of breakfast it is given sugar, which is easily broken down into glucose. Glucose is rapidly absorbed into the bloodstream and transported to the body's cells for either use or storage. By midmorning, the sugars have been digested, dispensed, and dissipated, leaving energy reserves low. The Blahs set in and you feel exhausted, have reduced attention span, and slowed physical and mechanical responses.

Unfortunately, what we often do when the Blahs hit is to reach for another sugar-filled food, causing the cycle to repeat. Instead we should eat more substantial foods. Whole wheat bread with peanut butter or cheese, and a piece of fruit and milk are as easy to carry along as a doughnut and coffee. Because they contain a mix of complex carbohydrates, fats and proteins, which are more slowly digested, energy level will be sustained without letdown.

The Blahs are a result of poor eating patterns. They should not be confused with hypoglycemia (low blood sugar) which results from a disorder of the pancreas causing it to secrete too much insulin, the hormone which regulates blood sugar levels. Several years ago, hypoglycemia was a popular self-diagnosis encouraged by fad diet books. It is a very rare disease which can only be diagnosed by laboratory tests. It is never a smart practice to decide on your own that you have a disease and then to proceed to treat yourself.

HONEY HIGHS

Rumors abound that some sugars are better than others. Not so! Honey, molasses, raw and unrefined brown sugars may taste better to you but to your body they are just sugar. They are not metabolized at a rate much different from white sugar. Neither do they contain significant amounts of any other nutrients. If trace minerals are present it is at such a low level that they do not make an important difference in your intake of that nutrient.

Furthermore, honest-to-goodness raw brown sugar is almost impossible to find today. Most of the brown sugar which you see in your grocery stores is refined white sugar which has either caramelized sugar or molasses added to it to give it color.

FABULOUS FRUCTOSE

Food manufacturers began adding corn sweetener and fructose to products instead of sugar in the mid-1970s when prices increased drastically for both cane and beet sugars. The substitution of corn sweetener went unnoticed. The addition of fructose was accompanied by claims that fructose is "the natural sweetener," the "type of sugar found in fruits and honey," and that it is "one and one half times as sweet as sugar."

Fructose does occur naturally in fruits and honey, so it is the same "type of sugar." However, the fructose added to our foods is not made from fruit. Granulated fructose is made by chemically splitting white sugar (sucrose) into its two component sugars, glucose and fructose, and then separating out the fructose. Liquid fructose is produced by treating corn syrup with enzymes to convert some of it to fructose. Therefore it is not extracted from fruits and is no more or less "natural" than sugars made from cane or beets.

"Fabulous fructose" diet claims promised us the same sweetness for less calories. Fructose has the same number of calories as any other sugar. It does have more sweetening power than regular sugar so less can be used. However, fructose tastes sweeter than sugar only in cold drinks and foods. For this reason, soft drink manufacturers seized upon fructose use to make "lite" colas. In foods which are served hot or at room temperature, such as baked goods, fructose is comparable to sugar in sweetness.

Finally, claims were made that fructose was somehow better for you because it is metabolized differently than sugar. It is metabolized slightly slower than sugar and does seem to require slightly less insulin. So it does have a less drastic fluctuation effect on blood sugar levels. Fructose may offer some slight advantages over other sugars, but it is still, first and foremost, a sugar which contains no nutrients other than calories.

PSEUDOSWEETS

Sugarholics in search of low-calorie, sweet foods and beverages have turned to sugar substitutes in an effort to control their weight, although there is no scientific evidence that it helps them to do so. The National Academy of Sciences estimates that 50 to 70 million Americans are "fairly regular" users of saccharin, including one-third of the nation's children under the age of 10. Two other artificial sweeteners, also called nonnutritive sweeteners because they contain neither calories nor vitamins nor minerals, are cyclamate and aspartame.

Saccharin, discovered in 1879, is manufactured from petroleum materials. So are plastic and gasoline. It is 300 times sweeter than sugar and has a slightly bitter aftertaste. There is some evidence that laboratory rats fed large quantities of saccharin will develop bladder cancer. The cancer-causing effects of saccharin, in humans, if any, are not conclusive.

A 1980 National Cancer Institute study of 9000 people found no general risks from use of artificial sweeteners. However, the researchers did conclude that heavy users of diet sodas and sugar substitutes and heavy smokers who also used artificial sweeteners, especially women, have a greater risk of bladder cancer than those who never use them. The institute also warned against use by nondiabetic children and pregnant women.

Cyclamate was banned by the FDA in 1970 when it was found to cause cancer in laboratory rats. It is thirty times sweeter than sugar, and until it was banned, was used in combination with saccharin and other sweeteners to enhance their sweetness.

The newest artificial sweetener is aspartame. It is made from protein and is digested like a protein in the body. Aspartame is 200 times sweeter than sugar and has been approved by the FDA for use in soft drinks and food and in granular form as a tabletop sweetener.

It is sold to consumers under the name Equal and to food manufacturers under the name NutraSweet. Its major disadvantage is that it decomposes under prolonged and high heat, so that it cannot be used in baking, and it gradually breaks down in liquids (soft drinks) which limits the time a product can sit on the grocery shelf.

One other group of substitute sweeteners exists, the polyalcohols: sorbitol, mannitol, and xylitol, used commonly in sugar-free chewing gum and special dietary foods for diabetics. Sorbitol and xylitol are absorbed more slowly than sugars but have the same number of calories as sugar. Thus a product made with them is "sugar-free" but not "calorie-free."

Mannitol is poorly absorbed and therefore supplies about half the number of calories as sugar does. Used in large amounts, greater than 20–50 grams per day, sorbitol and mannitol have a laxative effect.

Complex Carbohydrates

Starches such as potatoes, pasta, rice, whole grain products, and legumes are enjoying a new vogue. Starches were once avoided as "fattening," but today bookstores bulge with diets for pasta lovers, carbohydrate cravers, and rice-eating runners.

Complex carbohydrates are long chains of simple sugars strung together. To release the energy locked in them, the body must first break them down into their simple sugar components. It next converts these simple sugars to glucose, the form which body cells absorb and use for energy.

This entire process takes much longer than is required to absorb and metabolize the simple sugars, honey, fructose, and other refined sugars. For this reason, complex carbohydrate foods give a more even, constant, and sustained blood sugar level than simple sugars do. This slow energy release deters the "Blahs." See graph.

COMPARATIVE BLOOD SUGAR LEVELS

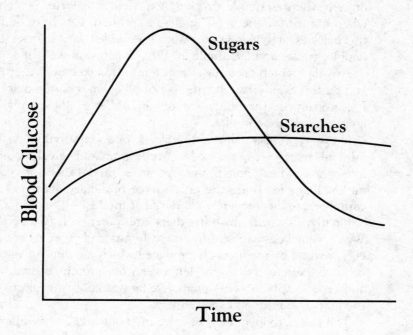

SOURCE: "Theory vs. Fact: The Glycemic Response to Foods," by Phyllis A. Crapo, R.D., *Nutrition Today*, March/April 1984.

A sustained energy supply is only one advantage of complex carbohydrates. Equally important is that they contain other essential vitamins and minerals, some protein, and very little, if any, fat.

A medium, whole, baked sweet potato contains 155 calories, 2 grams of protein, and almost twice the amount of vitamin A needed daily. A baked white potato contains 90 calories, and offers 3 grams of protein and one-third of the daily vitamin C requirements, in addition to smaller amounts of other nutrients.

THE "OLD" CARBOHYDRATE DIETS

Why would anyone think that carbohydrates are fattening and go on a low carbohydrate diet to lose weight?

We often laden starch foods with fats. We all love butter on our yams, sour cream on our baked potato, mayonnaise on our sandwich bread, and margarine on our toast. The starch food, without this added fat, is relatively low in calories. Carbohydrates, whether simple or complex, yield 4 calories per gram when burned for energy. The same as protein. Fats have double the calories at 9 per gram. With the added fat, calories can double, triple, and quadruple quickly, as can your waistline.

Any diet which takes away your toast also takes away your jam and butter. Sour cream by the spoonful becomes boring quickly. It is no surprise that a low-carbohydrate diet would sharply decrease your calorie intake.

However, it also reduces your intake of essential vitamins and minerals which are contained in whole grain and cereal products like whole wheat bread, rice, potatoes, and fruits and vegetables. Plant foods are the only source of dietary fiber, so low-carbohydrate diets severely restrict fiber intake.

Finally, low-carbohydrate diets are potentially dangerous. When your body is burning primarily fats and proteins for energy, several by-products are produced which are difficult for the body to excrete. Nitrogen, left over from protein breakdown, and ketones, products of incomplete fat breakdown, begin to tax the kidney's ability to excrete them.

The low-carbohydrate diet craze died quickly. It was unappetizing, results didn't last, and it was potentially dangerous. My husband also notes that it drove friends away because it made your breath smell bad!

THE "NEW" CARBOHYDRATE DIETS

The new carbohydrate diets stress foods high in complex carbohydrates. In truth these "new" diets are really a return to the way our grandmothers ate. In her heyday, Granny's diet had more whole grain cereals and products, dried beans, lentils, and peas than today's diet does.

Over the years we have replaced whole grain products with highly refined ones which are often loaded with sugar. Our intake of cakes, cookies, and bakery-type snack foods filled with sugary goo has gradually crept upward. We have replaced stone-cut oats with sugar-coated puffed oats at breakfast and baked potatoes at dinner with instant mashed potato flakes.

Not only have we changed the type, we have also decreased the total amount of carbohydrates we eat. Currently only about 45 percent of the calories in our diets are from carbohydrates. For Granny, between 60–65 percent of calories were from carbohydrates.

Experts recommend today that we return to Granny's eating habits: more complex carbohydrates, fewer simple ones, and less protein and fat. They encourage us to get up to 60 percent of our calories from starchy, fiber-filled foods. It's the "new" "old" diet: a return to plain and whole products, without added fats or sugars and with high fiber and nutrients.

There is increasing evidence suggesting that this "new" "old" type of eating will decrease the risk of heart disease and some cancers. In countries where as much as 70–80 percent of the calories come from whole grain and cereal foods and starchy vegetables, the incidence of heart and circulatory diseases is drastically lower than in the United States. Japanese, Italians, and Chinese rarely suffer with these diseases.

Fiber

Fiber is a calorie-free complex carbohydrate. It is undigestible. It passes through our digestive tract without breaking down. It is not really "essential" the way vitamins and minerals are. But you will see that it is nonetheless very important in our diet.

Our grandmothers called it "bulk" or "roughage" and made sure that they ate enough of it to keep "regular." Our mothers took diet pills filled with methylcellulose, a fiber, and ate diet breads made with wood pulp, all promising to "fill them up not out."

There are two major types of fiber: those that dissolve in hot water and those that are insoluble. Cellulose, hemicellulose, and lignin come from plant wall cells. They absorb water and therefore increase fecal bulk, which speeds the movement of food through the digestive tract, contributing to regularity. It's because of this that fiber fights constipation and diverticulosis.

Some scientists believe that eating high-fiber foods will prevent or control cancer, irritable bowel syndrome, and ulcerative colitis. There is no concrete evidence to confirm this but it looks highly probable.

Food fibers that dissolve in water form a pasty gel which delays absorption of other nutrients and slows the movement of food through the body. There is evidence that soluble fiber may help lower blood cholesterol levels. Soluble fibers include gums, mucilages, pectins, and storage polysaccharides. It is important to include some of each type of dietary fiber in your diet daily. Many foods which are excellent sources of one type of fiber will also be a good source of others. (See table 2.3.)

TABLE 2.3 TYPES OF FIBER

Insoluble		Soluble		
Cellulose	*Hemicellulose*	*Lignin*	*Gum*	*Pectin*
Apples	Beet root	Bran	Dried	Apples
Bran	Bran	Breakfast	beans	Cabbage
Broccoli	Brussels	cereals	Oatmeal	Carrots
Brussels sprouts	sprouts	Eggplant		Cauliflower
Cabbage	Cereals	Green		Citrus fruits
Carrots	Mustard	beans		Dried peas
Green beans	greens	Pears		Potatoes
Peppers	Whole	Radishes		Squash
Wax beans	grains			Strawberries
Whole wheat flour				

Insoluble—fibers absorb water; add bulk to stool; speed bowel movement; prevent constipation; may protect against colon cancer, diverticulosis, irritable bowel syndrome, and colitis	*Soluble*—fibers hold water; slow absorption of some nutrients; lower cholesterol level

Among the best news is that a diet high in fiber may be useful for weight reduction. Studies suggest that fruits, vegetables, and whole grains, all high in fiber and complex carbohydrates, are more satisfying to the appetite than diets high in fats and sugars. A high-fiber diet is also lower in calories, since fiber is not digested. It takes up space in the stomach. It absorbs water and slows down digestion to make you feel full longer.

Fiber is definitely the food for the fit generation. *The American Cancer Society* and the *National Cancer Institute* encourage us to eat more foods naturally high in fiber because of their potential benefits in reducing digestive system cancers. The *American Heart Association* and government agencies advise more fiber to reduce calorie intake and possibly decrease blood cholesterol levels. And if for no other reason, you should eat high-fiber foods to cut down on the purchase of laxatives!

How much we need is not clear. The average American now eats 10–20 grams a day. Researchers recommend that we increase that amount to above 30 grams. Some rural African people, who have much lower rates of heart disease, colon cancer, and diabetes than we do, eat over 60 grams daily.

Don't go overboard. As with anything good or bad, too much

can cause problems. Eating bran by the box isn't healthy. Too much can cause gas, bloating, and diarrhea. Excessive fiber can interfere with absorption of important minerals such as zinc, iron, calcium, and magnesium. Stick to a varied and balanced diet, selecting foods from the chart on opposite page.

Alcohol

Like carbohydrates, alcohol is composed of carbon, oxygen, and hydrogen molecules. Alcoholic beverages offer little in nutritive value. They yield about 7 calories per gram, slightly more than other carbohydrates, and contain trace amounts of B vitamins (niacin and thiamine) and iron.

Alcohol contributes about 5 percent of the calories in the average American diet. Consumption of beer and wine has increased over the past decade while use of hard liquors, such as gin, brandy, and bourbon, has decreased. In 1980 we drank 455 million gallons of hard liquor and 475.8 million gallons of wine.

Like all spirits, alcohol must be treated with respect. Abusive use is definitely dangerous. Drinking excessive amounts of alcohol can damage your brain, heart, and liver, irritate your stomach, and put stress on your kidneys.

When you drink, alcohol is sent directly to your liver where it is treated like a poison. The liver will detoxify the alcohol and then burn it for energy. Too much alcohol can damage the liver's ability to act as the body's poison clearinghouse.

Alcohol is a diuretic which increases your kidney's output of fluids and causes you to be thirsty and dry. This is why your mouth on the morning after too much booze feels like the Sahara after a pack of camels has trudged through.

Alcohol "loosens lips" and other inhibitions by deadening the brain's reasoning center. Excessive alcohol will further affect the brain, causing the slurred speech, stumbling stance, and blurred and confused vision of the drunk.

Laws passed in several states recently require that establishments selling alcoholic beverages must post warnings to pregnant women. Research studies of women who drank heavily during pregnancy showed an increase risk of physical abnormalities and mental retardation among their babies. The studies are not conclusive, but it certainly is not worth the risk to your baby's future to overindulge during your pregnancy.

Most doctors agree that total abstinence is best during the first three months of pregnancy when the baby is undergoing most of its critical development. Thereafter, an occasional drink is permissible. Caution is the best advice.

For those without the blush of pregnancy, small amounts of alcohol may offer some benefits. Nursing homes and hospitals often prescribe a small glass of sherry before dinner for elderly patients as an appetite stimulant. A little glass of Dubonnet with a twist will also get the digestive juices flowing!

My grandfather daily took his two jiggers of blackberry brandy. When we begged for sips, he would refuse us, claiming that it was his "heart medicine" and not for children! He may have been right. Recent studies suggest that moderate drinkers who consume one or two drinks daily live longer than those who refuse all alcohol or those who drink heavily. (Grandpa died at 94—not from heart failure.) Moderate amounts of alcohol raise the level of a protein (called high density lipoprotein or HDL) which binds fats and helps to reduce the level of fats in the blood and the accumulation of fats on the arterial walls. This reduces the risk of heart and arterial disease.

According to the U.S. Dietary Guidelines, a "moderate" amount is one to two drinks a day. Different drinks have different amounts of alcohol and therefore different amounts of calories. Table 2.4 lists serving sizes which provide 0.5 ounces of absolute alcohol—the amount which researchers use as one drink.

When I was a doctoral candidate in nutrition sciences at University of California, Berkeley, we graduate students met every Wednesday for discussions of highly technical aspects of current research. These sessions were occasionally followed by cookies and "punch." The punch was a blend of alcohol—pure stuff!— which we used in our studies, mixed with fruit juices. Not the best of blends but a cheap substitute for struggling student budgets!

Proteins

Real men don't eat quiche, but they do eat steak and potatoes. Steak builds men. Steak built America! At least, that seems to be the myth.

Countries in which the people eat more meat do seem to fare better economically. But to claim a connection is to put the cart before the cow. As countries become more affluent, they tend to

TABLE 2.4 CALORIES IN ALCOHOL

One Drink	Serving Size	Calories
Regular beers	12 oz	140–170
"Light" beers	12 oz	70–135
Sweet sherry	2 oz	95
Dry red wines	4 oz	85
Dry white wines	4 oz	80
"Light" white wines	4 oz	60

increase the amount of meat they eat. As we will see, this may not be necessary or beneficial.

All living tissue—whether plant or animal—contains protein. Proteins are the major building blocks of muscles, tendons, skin, hair, nails, and other tissues. They are also the main constituents of hemoglobin which binds and carries oxygen in the blood, of enzymes and hormones which regulate body functions, of antibodies which fight off infection, and of nucleic acids which carry the genetic codes or instructions for our bodies to grow and repair themselves. They are clearly pretty important.

Proteins, like carbohydrates, are chemically composed of carbon, oxygen, and hydrogen strung together in a chain. In addition, protein contains the chemical nitrogen. The presence of nitrogen distinguishes protein from fats and carbohydrates.

$$
\begin{array}{ccc}
H & H & O \\
\diagdown & \diagdown & \diagup \\
N & - C - C & \\
\diagup & \diagup & \diagdown \\
H & H & OH \\
\end{array}
\qquad \text{the amino acid, glycine}
$$

The nitrogen also allows chains to be linked together to form complicated patterns, like Chinese writing characters. Each "character" (a group of C-H-O-N) is called an amino acid. Proteins can contain hundreds of amino acids linked together just like a story contains many words or characters. An almost endless variety of stories are possible, depending on how the words are strung together. So it is with proteins.

The body can both break proteins into their component amino acids and manufacture proteins from amino acids. It can also manufacture some—but not all—amino acids from scratch. Those amino acids which it cannot make, but which it needs, are called "essential amino acids." They must be supplied to the body through the diet.

We need "enough" protein and the "right types." Protein cannot be stored by the body. Carbohydrates and fats can. When we eat more protein than we need, we simply break it down by removing the nitrogen and using the remaining C-H-O as if it were just another energy source. The nitrogen is excreted in the urine.

If protein is in short supply the body can make protein. Assuming that there are enough C-H-Os around from fats and carbohydrates to meet the body's energy needs, the body will recycle and reuse nitrogen to manufacture new proteins.

Because proteins are the body's building blocks, it will burn them for energy only if the body is short of calories from other sources. It spares protein, burning it only as a last resort.

When you go on a diet to lose weight and eat less calories than your body needs, your body will burn your body fat for fuel before it will use muscle or other protein tissues. When it runs out of fat, it will burn muscle and other protein tissue. Anorexics, underfed prisoners of war, those suffering from hunger, and people on unbalanced, severely low-calorie diets to lose weight, can lose hair and muscle tissue.

Except for self-imposed low-protein diets, a deficient intake of protein is very rare in America. In fact, we eat more protein than is necessary to maintain our health. We need only about 12 percent of our calories as protein. Currently approximately 18–20 percent of the calories in the average diet comes from protein foods. That's about 6 ounces of steak or almost half of a chicken—definitely manhandler-size portions.

By nature, animal proteins come packaged with fat. So as our protein intake has increased, so has our intake of fats. And as you will discover in the section on fats which follows this, animal fats in excess may have harmful consequences for our health.

In the past decades, concerned with high protein and fat intakes, many Americans have cut back on meat intake and others have given it up altogether, becoming vegetarians. Is it safe to cut back, and if so, how much protein is enough?

Animal proteins, meats, fish, poultry, dairy products, and eggs, are "complete" proteins. That is, they contain a good supply of all of the essential amino acids—those which our body cannot manufacture and must therefore get from the diet. When we include animal protein foods in our diets, the essential amino acids are supplied.

Plant foods, vegetables, grains and cereals, beans and legumes, also contain protein. However, they contain larger amounts of complex carbohydrate and fiber. So we don't tend to think of them as sources of protein. Plant foods are often low in one or more essential amino acids. Fortunately, they are not all low in the same amino acids. So it is possible to eat a combination of plant foods that will provide a complete complement of essential amino acids.

These combinations are called complementary proteins. Many of our favorite ethnic dishes are complementary plant protein combinations. Mexican tortillas and frijoles (corn and beans), Italian pasta fagioli (wheat and beans), Chinese rice with tofu (soybeans), and all-American peanut butter on whole wheat bread provide all the essential amino acids which your body needs.

Strict vegetarians who eat no animal products supply their body's need for essential amino acids from combination/complementary dishes like these. Vegetarians who include some dairy products and eggs in their diet (called lacto-ovo vegetarians) are assured sufficient essential amino acids.

Plant sources of protein are considerably less expensive than animal sources as shown in table 2.5. All the essential amino acids are supplied by the combinations listed. Note that the amount of protein and fat in each choice is also listed. Generally, plant proteins contain considerably less fat than animal sources of protein.

Americans, Australians, and Argentineans—all residents of major cattle countries—eat considerably more meat than the rest of the world. Restaurant menus boast steaks served in your

TABLE 2.5 PROTEIN COMPARISONS

Dish	Portion	Amount Protein (g)	Amount Fat (g)	Cost
Steak, lean and fat	3 oz	20	27	75¢
Pork chop, loin	3 oz	21	24	53¢
Egg omelet	3 eggs and 1 tbsp butter	18	30	31¢
Beans and cornbread	1 cup 1 muffin	18	5	8¢
Black-eyed peas and rice	1 cup 1 cup	17	1	9¢

Source: Values from USDA Home and Garden Bulletin, No. 72, 1978.

choice of 12-, 14-, or 16-ounce portions and quarter-pound hamburgers with cheese.

For most of the world's citizens, animal proteins are used as a condiment to complement and complete vegetable proteins. In India, a half pound of meat served with rice, lentils, and vegetables will provide adequate protein for a family of four to six members.

The richest and most complete sources of plant proteins are legumes—dried peas, lentils, and beans of all types—kidney, pinto, black, red (not green beans), limas, and soybeans. Vegetarians depend upon these foods for their daily protein needs.

Tofu, a curd made from soybeans, closely resembles animal proteins. It is a mainstay of Asian diets and is becoming more popular in America because of its versatility and low cost. In addition to its many main-dish uses, it is even made into a low-fat, ice-cream-type dessert called Tofutti.

Nuts, seeds such as sesame and sunflower, and peanuts are good plant protein sources. These foods are generally a bit more expensive than dried beans and peas—but still a bargain when compared to meat prices. They also contain fat, which beans and peas do not. A Chinese dish of stir-fried broccoli with water chestnuts and cashews over rice provides complete amino acids. So does the Middle Eastern dish hommos (made from chickpeas) served over couscous, a type of wheat.

Other plant foods also contain protein, but not in sufficient amount to consider them primary protein providers.

When we add up the protein from all the sources in our diet, it is surprising to see how much we actually eat. We can begin to see places where we could cut back or substitute less costly proteins.

Animal proteins contain a good share of fat—sometimes as much as 80 percent of the calories (table 2.6). By substituting plant protein for some of the animal protein in our meals, we can cut calories, cost, and fat.

Table 2.7 is a typical day's menu for the "average" American male. It contains 93 grams of protein. That's more than one and one-half times the approximately 60 grams of protein that an adult male needs.

Experts agree that we should cut back our protein intake, decreasing the proportional amount of protein in our meals to 12–15 percent of calories. Table 2.8 gives an example of how to do this. Notice that the quantity of food remains about the same

TABLE 2.6 PERCENT CALORIES FROM FAT IN PROTEIN FOODS

Dish	Portion	Total Calories per portion	Calories from Fat	Percent Calories from Fat
Steak	3 oz	330	243	74
Pork chop	3 oz	310	216	70
Egg omelet	3 eggs and 1 tbsp butter	340	270	79
Beans and cornbread	1 cup 1 muffin	355	45	13
Blackeyed peas and rice	1 cup 1 cup	415	9	2

Source: *USDA Bulletin*, No. 72.

TABLE 2.7 THE 93-GRAM PROTEIN MENU

Food	Serving	Calories	Protein (g)	Fat (g)
Eggs, poached	2	160	12	12
Toast, whole wheat	2	130	6	2
Butter, pat	1	35	tr[a]	4
Cheese sandwich				
Whole wheat bread	2	130	6	2
Cheddar cheese, 1 oz	2	330	14	18
Mayonnaise, tbsp	1	100	tr[a]	11
Milk, whole, cup	1	160	9	9
Apple, whole	1	70	tr[a]	tr[a]
Cookies, chocolate chip	3	150	3	9
Roast beef, 1 oz	5	625	28	56
Potatoes, mashed, cup	1	125	4	1
Broccoli, cup	1	40	5	1
Lettuce, head	1/4	10	1	tr[a]
Dressing, tbsp	1	65	tr[a]	6
Dinner roll	1	155	5	2
Butter, pat	1	35	tr[a]	4
Total		2320	93	137

[a] Trace amount.

but that the number of calories and the amount of total protein goes down when less animal protein is used.

Lower protein, lower fat menus are also lower in cost. The table 2.7 menu costs $2.62 per person. The table 2.8 menu saves calories, fat intake, and pennies at a cost of $2.02 per person.

TABLE 2.8 THE 66-GRAM PROTEIN MENU

Food	Serving	Calories	Protein (g)	Fat (g)
Oatmeal, cup	1	130	5	2
Whole milk, cup	¼	40	2	2
Banana	1	100	1	tr[a]
Toast, whole wheat	2	130	6	2
Butter, pat	1	35	tr[a]	4
Lunch sandwich				
Whole wheat bread	2	130	6	2
Peanut butter, tbsp	1	95	4	4
Jam, tbsp	1	55	tr[a]	tr[a]
Milk, whole, cup	1	160	9	9
Apple	1	70	tr[a]	tr[a]
Cookies, chocolate chip	3	150	3	9
Beef and vegetable				
stew, cup	1	210	15	10
Rice, cup	1	225	4	tr[a]
Broccoli, cup	1	40	5	1
Lettuce, head	¼	10	1	tr[a]
Dressing, tbsp	1	65	tr[a]	6
Dinner roll	1	155	5	2
Butter, pat	1	35	tr[a]	4
Total		1835	66	57

[a] Trace amount.

Fats

Fats are the body's warehouse of fuel, kept in storage until needed for energy when the food you eat fails to provide enough. When fats are burned they provide more than twice the energy as an equal amount of either protein or carbohydrates.

Body fat acts as insulation to keep the body temperature even.

There is a layer of fat below our outside skin surface which protects us from extremes of hot and cold. It is also a cushion against physical trauma to the body. All those little pads and pouches around your abdomen, hips, and joints protect vital organs and movable joints from injury. In babies, who frequently fall, fat cushions are concentrated around knees and elbows.

Fat in the body is inevitable and indispensable. Our body manufactures fat from excess calories. We do not need to eat fat in order to make fat. Therefore we need very little fat from our diet, only enough to ensure that we get the essential fatty acid, linoleic acid, and the fat-soluble vitamins, A, D, E, and K. Two other fatty acids, arachidonic and linolenic are sometimes called essential. Like linoleic, the body cannot manufacture them, so they must be provided from the diet.

A tablespoon of polyunsaturated oil—safflower, soybean, corn, or other vegetable oil, will provide you with all the essential fatty acid which you need. It can be provided even when less than 2 percent of total calories come from fats.

Most of us pad our fat intake and thereby pad our pants far too generously. We need only about 2 percent of calories as fat to supply our essential fatty acid needs, yet about 40 percent of our calories come from fat. Dietary fats provide 9 calories per gram as compared to 4 calories per gram from carbohydrates and protein. It is often our high fat intake which contributes to excess calorie intake.

When the body has accumulated 3500 extra calories, it stores a pound of body fat. It does not need to collect these calories all on the same day. We can gain a pound in a week by consuming 500–600 extra calories each day. To shed that pound of weight will require that you burn up 3500 calories.

Potential weight gain from concentrated fat calories is not the only risk. The amount and type of fat in our diet also have important health consequences. High fat intake, particularly high-saturated fat intake, contributes to elevated levels of fats in the blood. Elevated blood fat levels increase the risk of heart disease, stroke, and other arterial diseases.

What's in a Fat?

Fats are composed of the elements carbon and hydrogen strung together in chains. Each chain is called a fatty acid. Whether a fatty acid is saturated or not depends on the number of hydrogen atoms connected to each carbon. When the carbon chain con-

tains as many hydrogen atoms as it will hold, it is called "saturated."

```
    H   H   H   H   H
     \   \   \   \   \
  H — C — C — C — C — C — H
     /   /   /   /   /
    H   H   H   H   H
```

Saturated fats are solid or semisolid at room temperature. The
layer of fat on the edge of your steak, fat in chicken skin, and
the marbling of a piece of lamb, which are all firm and visible at
room temperature, are saturated fats.

Fats are not 100 percent saturated or unsaturated. They contain some of each. The percentage contained will determine how
solid they are. Butter is 57 percent saturated fat, margarines are
23 percent saturated. At room temperature, butter will be soft
but will hold its stick form. Margarine will melt and lose its
form.

Monounsaturated and unsaturated fats contain less hydrogen
than they could. Some of the carbon atoms in these fats form
double bonds to one another rather than attaching to a hydrogen.

```
    H   H   H   H   H   H
     \   \   \   \   \   \
  H — C — C — C = C — C — C — H
     /   /           /   /
    H   H           H   H
```

Polyunsaturated fats have more than one double bond. These
fats are liquid at room temperature and are called oils.

```
    H   H   H   H   H   H   H
     \   \   \   \   \       \
  H — C — C = C — C = C = C — C — H
     /                       /
    H                       H
```

Fatty acids found in vegetables tend to be monounsaturated,
unsaturated, or polyunsaturated. Some margarines and cooking
shortenings are made from vegetable oils. To give them a firmer
consistency, manufacturers will chemically break open double
carbon bonds to add hydrogen. When this has been done, the
ingredient label will read "hydrogenated vegetable oil added."

This will increase saturation and the fat will no longer be an oil at room temperature.

Certain oils, such as coconut oil, palm oil, and cocoa butter contain high levels of saturated fatty acids, even though they are plant fats. They are used frequently in coffee creamers, processed foods, and imitation dairy products. They offer no nutritional advantages over cream or butter fats.

Because of the important health consequences of fat, food labels may advertise which type of fat the product contains or does not contain. The words "a polyunsaturated oil," "contains no saturated fat," or "cholesterol free" are common today.

Diseases Related to Fat

Cardiovascular diseases, which include heart attacks and strokes, cause more deaths in the United States than all causes of death combined, including cancer. Underlying this disease is a condition called atherosclerosis, the accumulation of fatty debris in the arteries, which causes them to narrow and harden. Blood passage becomes restricted causing increased blood pressure. If a passage to the brain becomes completely blocked, stroke occurs. If a passage to the heart becomes blocked, heart attack results.

The causes of atherosclerotic diseases are many. High levels of cholesterol in the blood, high-fat diets, smoking, too little exercise, and possibly a stressful personality, all contribute.

Until recently, the exact role of high-fat, high-cholesterol diets was debated. A study of over 3000 subjects conducted by the National Heart, Lung and Blood Institute, released in 1984, ended the debate. Diets high in fat are associated with high levels of blood cholesterol and lowering blood cholesterol will reduce the risk of heart disease.

Calories and Fat

Reducing fat intake can be difficult because not all fats are visible. One gram of fat supplies about 9 calories, twice the amount found in carbohydrates or protein. It is important to know where fat is hidden. Table 2.9 groups foods by the percentage of calories in that food which comes from fat.

Cholesterol Controversy

Cholesterol is a waxy fat found in all body cells. It is essential to the health of body cell walls, and is used to make vitamin D and several hormones, including sex hormones. Our bodies have the

TABLE 2.9 PERCENTAGE OF CALORIES FROM FAT IN COMMON FOODS

Percent	Foods
More than 90%	Bacon, mayonnaise, butter, margarine, salad and cooking oil, lard, cream, baking chocolate, vegetable shortening
80–90%	Sausages, most salad dressings, corned beef, cream cheese, unsweetened coconut, walnuts, pecans, sesame seeds
65–80%	Potato chips, dry toasted peanuts, ham, frankfurters, American cheese, Swiss cheese, Cheddar cheese, sunflower seeds, cashews, peanut butter
50–65%	Broiled beef-loin steaks, roasted leg of lamb
35–50%	Most cookies, crackers, cakes, and doughnuts, round steak, lean ground beef, whole milk
20–35%	Low-fat (2%) milk
10–20%	Roasted chicken (without skin), broiled fish
Negligible	Skim milk, dry cereal, dry cottage cheese (no added milk fat), dried beans, baked or boiled potatoes, most breads, fruits, and vegetables (except avocados and olives)

Source: Michigan Department of Public Health, 1980.

ability to manufacture cholesterol, so there is no need to get cholesterol from the food we eat.

Cholesterol circulates in the blood whether or not our diets contain cholesterol. The average American's circulating cholesterol level is between 225–250 milligrams per 100 milliliters of blood serum. Many experts in the field believe that this is too high. In countries with very low incidence of atherosclerosis, blood cholesterol levels average between 150–175.

Blood cholesterol is easy to measure. At your next physical examination, ask your doctor to draw a blood sample and have it measured. If your level is above 200 milligrams you can benefit from cutting back your intake of saturated fats and cholesterol. There are individuals who have diets low in cholesterol but who nonetheless have high blood cholesterol levels due to their body's own manufacturing of cholesterol. Generally, however, if your levels are high it is because your intakes are high.

Cholesterol is carried throughout the body by a chemical called a lipoprotein. There are three types of carriers: high-density lipoproteins (HDLs), low density lipoproteins (LDLs), and very-low-density lipoproteins (VLDLs). LDLs and VLDLs deposit cholesterol in the cells and arteries. HDLs return choles-terol to the liver where it is turned into bile and excreted by the intestines.

People with high levels of HDLs have lower circulating levels of cholesterol in their bloods. They suffer less from artery dis-eases and less frequently die of heart attacks or stroke. Aerobic exercises such as strenuous exercise, jogging, long-distance run-ning, and bicycling will increase HDLs. Changing the propor-tion of saturated to polyunsaturated fats in your diet to favor the polyunsaturated may also increase HDLs.

The American Heart Association recommends that daily in-takes of cholesterol for ALL people not exceed 300 milligrams. Most of us eat around 600 milligrams of cholesterol daily. From table 2.10, it is clear that some foods are very high in cholesterol content. These foods—eggs, red meat, etc.—should be eaten in moderation.

Diets high in saturated fats also raise blood cholesterol level. Fortunately, the same foods which are high in cholesterol are high in saturated fats, so that limiting the amount of one also controls the amount of the other.

Polyunsaturated fats do not raise blood cholesterol level and do not increase the risk of heart disease. Some questions have been raised about whether or not they may contribute to cancer, particularly colon cancer. Several animal studies have suggested that they might. However, there is no increased incidence of cancers among Japanese whose dietary fat is predominantly poly-unsaturated fats from vegetable oils.

Cancer and Fat

Colon, breast, and endometrium cancers do seem to occur more frequently in people who eat diets high in total fat. The mecha-nisms by which fat increases the rate of these cancers are not yet clear. It is clear that people who eat low-fat diets have a lower risk of these cancers.

The recommended level of fats in our diets is not more than 30 percent of total calories. The menus in chapter 4 give exam-ples of how to cut fat without cutting pleasure.

Vitamins

Vitamins are substances essential to our health and which our bodies cannot manufacture. Like essential amino acids and es-

TABLE 2.10 FATTY ACID AND CHOLESTEROL CONTENT OF COMMON MEASURES OF SELECTED FOODS

Food	Amount	% Fat (by wt)	Choles-terol (mg)	Calories
Vegetable oils: safflower, soybean, corn, sesame, etc.	1 tbsp	97	0	120
Milk, nonfat, skim, fluid	1 cup	0	5	90
Cottage cheese, low-fat	½ cup	1	5	82
Cottage cheese, creamed, small curd	½ cup	4.5	15	108
Ice cream, regular	½ cup	10.7	30	134
Cheese, Cheddar	1 oz	33.6	30	114
Milk, whole, fluid	1 cup	3.3	33	150
Butter	1 tbsp	81	31	102
Oysters, Eastern, raw	3 oz	2	42	56
Chicken, light meat, without skin	3 oz	4.4	72	147
Chicken, light meat, fried with skin	3 oz	12	74	209
Beef, rib roast, lean and fat, roasted	3 oz	33	70	330
Beef, ground, cooked well done	3 oz	18	88	244
Lamb, lean only	3 oz	1	80	183
Shrimp, dry-pack, canned	3 oz	1	128	99
Egg, whole or yolk	1	11	274	79
Beef liver, fried	3 oz	10.5	372	195

Source: USDA, *Provisional Table on the Fatty Acid and Cholesterol Content of Selected Foods*, June 1984.

sential fatty acid, we must get them from the foods we eat. They do not provide energy, nor do they construct or build any part of the body.

Without vitamins, we cannot use the foods we eat for energy, building and repairing our bodies, or other processes which are essential to life. They have critical roles at each step of the process through which foodstuffs are metabolized. If a key vitamin is missing at any one of the steps, metabolism cannot continue, even though everything else required is present. Cells could actually starve in a sea of available nutrients when a critical vitamin is missing.

The result of a deficiency can be tissues which cease to grow and develop or repair themselves. Sores, rashes, dizziness, fatigue, fuzzy thinking, blurred vision, and other symptoms may occur. Generally these symptoms will occur in groups and are called "syndromes."

Vitamin deficiency syndromes can look like syndromes caused by other disease problems. You should not self-diagnose or depend upon the judgment and advice of an untrained person, such as a vitamin store sales clerk. If symptoms occur and persist, see a qualified physician who can differentiate symptoms and causes and prescribe appropriate treatment.

There are 13 recognized vitamins. Most of them are water-soluble and carried by the blood throughout the body. Excesses of these vitamins are washed out of the body through the urine and sweat. They are not stored so must be constantly resupplied by the diet.

Because they are water-soluble, they can also be washed out of our foods. Most of them are easily destroyed by heat and air exposure.

Four of the vitamins are not soluble in water. They are fat-soluble and are absorbed along with fats in the diet. They are resistant to water and cannot be washed out of the body. They are stored in the body's fat storage warehouses. We do not have to eat fat-soluble vitamins daily. And if we take in an excess of these vitamins, they can accumulate to toxic levels.

There are several other substances which some claim to be vitamins. These are not recognized by the scientists who set standards for the Recommended Dietary Allowances. To be called a vitamin, a chemical has to meet strict criteria: it must be organic (minerals are not vitamins), it must be essential to some bodily functions, and absence from the diet must result in specific defects.

"Nonvitamins" which you may see in health food and drug-stores include choline, inositol, Laetrile (called vitamin B-17, promoted as a cancer cure), pangamic acid (vitamin B-15), PABA (para-aminobenzoic acid, a good sunscreen only), and rutin (which is essential for crickets but not for people).

Research is far from final. The first vitamins were isolated in the early 1900s. The possibility exists that others will be discovered. And certainly we are daily learning more about the intricacies, interactions, and actions of those vitamins which are already recognized.

Following is a table of brief descriptions of each of the 13 vitamins, their role in our health, symptoms of deficiency and over or megadoses, and important food sources of each. Important current issues or controversies are covered in the text along with accounts of some unusual experiences with patients.

The Fat-Soluble Vitamins

VITAMIN A

At one time, vitamin A was prescribed by dermatologists for skin problems such as acne and pimples. Its usefulness in preventing or curing these problems was found to be limited and it is no longer routinely prescribed.

A chemical compound very similar in structure to vitamin A, called Acutane, is being tested for use with severe skin infections and disorders. It is given in massive doses and is not vitamin A.

More recently vitamin A has come into vogue as a preventive or curative for cancer, particularly skin cancers. There is evidence that suggests that people with low vitamin A intakes do suffer more frequently from skin and other types of cancers. However, there is no evidence that intakes of vitamin A substantially above the recommended levels will either prevent or cure cancers.

Massive doses of vitamin A are toxic. It is a fat-soluble vitamin and will accumulate in the liver and the body's fat tissues. Toxic levels usually result from taking vitamin A supplements. It is difficult to get too much vitamin A from food.

Vitamin A is found only in animal foods—fish and beef liver, and eggs. Precursors of vitamin A, substances from which our bodies can synthesize vitamin A, are found widely in plant foods. Carotene, provitamin A, is found in dark green leafy vegetables and deep yellow-orange foods like carrots and apricots. The deeper the green or yellow-orange color, the more carotene present.

Carotene is nontoxic and will not result in toxicity symptoms if taken in excess. But it can produce symptoms. A nutritionist in Arizona reported to me that a patient in one of the county's health clinics came in because he had turned light yellow-orange in color. She suspected, and was right, that he was drinking massive quantities of carrot juice daily. This seems to be the only symptom of excess carotene intake.

VITAMIN D

The main job of the "sunshine" vitamin is to regulate calcium and phosphorous metabolism to build and maintain strong bones and teeth.

Food sources of vitamin D are limited. It was once popular to administer vile and viscous tablespoons of cod-liver oil to children during the winter to protect against rickets. Fortunately today our milk supply is fortified with vitamin D and it's much easier to swallow.

Most people get sufficient vitamin D by exposure to the sun. A provitamin or precursor of vitamin D found under the skin surface is transformed into D when sunlight hits it. As little as ten to fifteen minutes a day of noontime sun can provide more than enough vitamin D. A fat-soluble vitamin, D is stored and available during winter months when there is less sun.

Artificial light, light filtered through glass or smog, and exposure to sun without exposure of skin to direct rays will not do the job. With this fear in mind, a patient of mine in San Francisco took her two-month-old infant out on a rare sunny winter day for some vitamin D synthesis. Poor baby was sunburned from top to toe and cried miserably for several days. A little sun goes a long way on a little bottom!

VITAMIN E

Vitamin E has enjoyed two short-lived reputed careers: one as the "sex" vitamin and another as the "antiaging" drug. It was first discovered when it was noted that in the absence of this substance, laboratory rats became less fertile and productive and if pregnant, might resorb the fetuses. For this reason it was named tocopherol which means the ability to bear young.

In subsequent years, E enthusiasts claimed that the vitamin could cure impotency in men and increase fertility in women. This claim has never been verified and is discredited.

A popular book in the late sixties touted vitamin E as the preventive pill for heart disease. That too was an unfounded and short-lived claim.

More recently, vitamin E was consumed by those racing the clock, in the hopes of slowing the aging process.

Vitamin E is a powerful antioxidant which prevents oxygen from reacting with unsaturated fats in the body causing rancid decomposition. This deterioration process is similar to the aging process. There is evidence that vitamin E may delay this deterioration process in laboratory animals and live human tissues grown outside the body in laboratory cultures. None of the evidence is conclusive and it does not look hopeful for a Ponce de León pill.

Vitamin E is present in many plants including lettuce and

peanuts. Seed oils are an excellent source along with all vegetable oils. Generally the amount of E present parallels the amount of polyunsaturated fats present. This is fortunate. Our need for vitamin E increases as our intake of polyunsaturated fats increases.

VITAMIN K

Vitamin K is necessary for the normal clotting of blood. No myths or misuses have abounded with K. It is fairly widely distributed in small amounts throughout our food supply. It is synthesized by bacteria in our gut. Deficiencies rarely occur.

The Water-Soluble Vitamins

ASCORBIC ACID, VITAMIN C

Of all the vitamins, C enjoys the widest renown as miracle nutrient. It is consumed in massive doses, from 10 to 20 times recommended intakes, by persons who believe that it will cure the common cold, improve athletic performance, prevent infections in general, cure cancer, and a range of other promises.

Body tissues will become saturated with vitamin C when intakes exceed 100–150 milligrams daily. Thereafter, what goes in, comes out. You are simply flushing nutrients down the toilet.

When the famed Dr. Linus Pauling, a Nobel Prize Laureate, announced his book, *Vitamin C and the Common Cold,* we were sure that drippy noses, hackers' cough, and pulsing headaches were gone forever. Numerous studies of thousands of subjects have failed to verify his claim that vitamin C can prevent the common cold. It may minimize the symptoms but even this is not certain and may be a result of the user's belief that it will help rather than any actual help resulting from C use.

Notwithstanding scientific research, faithful followers still pop thousands of C tablets each winter and swear that they have fewer colds than before. There is no accounting for their claim. It may be like the blessing which Alan King was known to give when departing from the home of others: "May your house be safe from tigers." If you protested his silly blessing, saying that you had never seen a tiger in the neighborhood, he would respond that it was proof that his blessing was working. Neither is there scientific proof that megadoses of vitamin C can cure or prevent cancer, atherosclerotic or heart disease.

Bicyclists and other endurance athletes swear that vitamin C improves their performance and endurance. There is no evidence to support this claim. Interestingly, because of athletic interest in high C intakes, a fruit juice drink was given the name Hi-C.

Studies of smokers suggest that their needs for vitamin C may be higher than that of nonsmokers. However, their needs are not so high that they cannot be met from food sources and it is not necessary to take a supplement if you smoke. The first and best health measure would be to stop smoking. Failing that, make sure that you get at least a large glass of orange juice daily or one of the other C-rich foods.

In certain therapeutic situations, massive doses of C may be given as a drug or medicine. In these situations, C is no longer functioning as a nutrient but has taken on a pharmacological effect. Massive doses should not be self-prescribed or taken without medical supervision.

B VITAMINS

As a group the B vitamins are essential to the metabolism and release of energy of protein, carbohydrates, and fats. If B vitamins are lacking, energy metabolism is incomplete.

THIAMINE, VITAMIN B-1

As your carbohydrate intake increases, so does your need for thiamine. This presents a particular problem for those who eat large quantities of refined sugars, refined, unenriched cereal products, or alcohol. Thiamine intakes may be insufficient to meet the metabolic demands of these foods.

The solution is not more thiamine. Switch to more complex carbohydrate foods which are either unrefined or enriched. Milling and processing carbohydrates such as rice and wheat remove much of the thiamine. It is added back through enrichment. Sugars are not enriched. Neither are alcohols.

Unrefined complex carbohydrate foods, whole grain cereals and products contain thiamine in amounts sufficient to meet the body's needs in metabolizing the carbohydrate contained.

There is no validity to the claim that thiamine taken in excess doses will give your skin a smell or taste which will repel mosquitoes.

RIBOFLAVIN, VITAMIN B-2

Milk is the primary source of B-2. B-2 is easily destroyed by light. That's why our milk is no longer delivered to the doorstep in clear glass bottles. Dairy products are delivered now in opaque plastic or wax-covered cardboard containers to prevent B-2 loss.

NIACIN

Niacin does not cure schizophrenia, hyperactivity, childhood autism, alcoholism, arthritis, high blood cholesterol, neurosis, or depression. Its primary role is to participate in the release of energy from foods.

PYRIDOXINE, VITAMIN B-6

B-6 is essential to protein metabolism. As our intake of protein increases, so should our intake of B-6. Whole grains—unprocessed and unrefined—are the best source of B-6. It is lost from these foods during the milling process and may or may not be added back by enrichment.

COBALAMIN, VITAMIN B-12

B-12 shots are administered on a regular basis by some practitioners as a cure for depression, tiredness, and listlessness. There is no conclusive evidence that they work.

Strict vegetarians, those who eat no animal products, risk B-12 deficiencies. Plant foods do not contain B-12. Only animal foods do. Even yeasts, such as brewer's yeast, which are commonly taken as a "natural" source of B vitamins, contain no B-12. Many strict vegetarians take B-12 supplements.

FOLACIN, FOLIC ACID, OR FOLATE

In the past ten years, obstetricians have begun prescribing folate supplements for pregnant women. Demand for this nutrient is increased during pregnancy and it was feared that intakes of folic acid were low or marginal in the U.S. diet.

Oral supplements of folate are associated with a reduced risk of small-for-date births. For this reason, the National Academy of Sciences states that oral supplements appear desirable to maintain the mother's stores and keep pace with increased use of this vitamin during pregnancy.

Minerals

Minerals have become the new miracle supplements. Today we hear as much about zinc, calcium, and iron as we do about the vitamins.

Like vitamins, minerals are found throughout the body. They are components of hormones, enzymes, and of our hard body tissues, bones, and teeth. They also play a specific and critical role in water regulation, muscle contractions, and nerve cell transmissions.

Minerals in foods usually occur in combinations with one another or with organic compounds and are called salts. Sodium combined with chloride forms the mineral salt, sodium chloride, which we know as table salt. Potassium chloride, also a mineral salt, is used as a table salt substitute.

Each mineral carries a positive or negative electrical charge and follows the old adage that "opposites attract." Sodium has a positive charge and so it combines with chloride which has a negative charge. Potassium also has a positive charge and cannot combine with sodium to form a salt, but can combine with chloride.

The importance of all of this is that when these minerals dissolve in the water of our bodies, they can attract and repel each other. They are called "electrolytes" and play a major role in determining how much water our bodies retain or expel.

By interacting with one another, they cause muscles to relax and contract as if an electrical signal had been sent through them. And they make possible the transmission of currents through our nervous system. We need more of some minerals than of others. Calcium, chloride, magnesium, phosphorus, potassium, sodium, and sulfur are needed in large amounts, but not megadoses. We need only very small amounts of chromium, copper, fluoride, iodine, iron, manganese, molybdenum, selenium, and zinc, so these are called trace minerals.

You may see arsenic, cadmium, cobalt, nickel, and other minerals being sold in drug- and health food stores. At this time, these are not recognized by the National Academy of Sciences to be essential minerals.

The Water Regulators: Sodium, Potassium, Chloride

Our bodies are two-thirds water—about 40–50 quarts. Body fluids compose the major portion of body cells and the cells themselves float in fluid. The thin wall which surrounds the cells, the membrane, separates the water or fluid inside from that outside the cell.

The movement of fluid from inside to outside the cell and the reverse is controlled by the concentration of salts in the fluid on either side of the cell membrane. This is very critical. If the balance is upset we can lose too much fluid, becoming dehydrated, or retain too much fluid, becoming swollen and edemic.

Sodium is the key element outside the cell and potassium the key element inside the cell involved in the transfer of fluids. Chloride (remember it has a negative charge) combines with each of them to form their respective salts, sodium chloride and potassium chloride.

As the body's fluids pass through the kidney, at the rate of about one quart per minute, the kidney checks the concentration of salts. If the concentration is high, the kidney will excrete salts in the urine. If the concentration is low, the kidney will save the sodium and other salts and recirculate them through the body.

This mechanism fails in approximately one out of every five Americans, leading to a condition called hypertension. Two factors seem to contribute to hypertension: heredity and high salt intakes. Some people's kidneys just do not do a good job of sensing and regulating salt excretion. Other people, who have excessively high salt intakes, may overload and damage the kidney's ability to accurately detect and excrete salts.

When the kidney fails to excrete salts properly, they accumulate. They attract and hold water in an attempt to dilute themselves to a safe concentration. This increases both the volume of blood circulating and the amount of fluids in and around the cell. The body becomes waterlogged.

The tiny arteries which carry blood to the cells restrict in an attempt to stop drowning the cells with water. This causes blood to remain in the larger arteries where blood volume has already increased.

The heart tries to pump faster in order to move the increased volume of blood, and sends signals for the vessels to contract to slow down the blood flow. As the vicious cycle repeats and repeats, the pressure of all that fluid fighting for space climbs higher.

This condition is called high blood pressure or hypertension.

If it becomes too severe, congestive heart failure or stroke can follow. In congestive heart failure the heart simply cannot manage the increased volume of fluid and exhausts itself trying. In stroke, an artery or arteries in the brain explode from the pressure. Stroke may result in crippling of various body parts or death.

Other risk factors are involved in hypertension, and the above is a simplification. Yet it explains the essence of water regulation and the role played by mineral salts.

The body sometimes loses electrolytes too. During severe vomiting or diarrhea caused by flus and other infections, excess amounts of potassium and sodium may be lost. Diuretics, prescribed for hypertensive patients, obese persons, and used sometimes to alleviate the pressure of premenstrual cramps, can cause electrolyte loss. If loss continues for long periods of time or is severe, weakness, muscle cramps, and dehydration can occur.

Intense exercise, like running marathons, and intense physical work, especially if performed in the hot sun, can lead to excess sweating and electrolyte loss. Water losses over 4–5 pounds can result in leg cramps, dizziness, and headache. The crucial and immediate need is to replace the water lost through sweating.

There is no reason to take salt tablets. This was once a common practice but is no longer advised by sports nutritionists. Under extreme conditions, such as a marathon on a hot, humid day, electrolytes can be replaced by adding a small amount of salt to the water drunk, as little as one-quarter teaspoon per quart of water.

Your body alerts you when you need fluids. You become thirsty. That's why a cold beer tastes so good at a picnic when it's hot out and you have been playing ball and eating salty chips all afternoon. It is also why bars serve free pretzels, peanuts, and beer nuts!

SODIUM

Sodium enters our diet through table salt and in various chemicals used in food preservation and processing. About one-fourth of the sodium we eat is as sodium chloride, table salt, which we add at the stove or the table. Another fourth occurs naturally in foods which are high in sodium—milk and celery are examples.

The remaining half is added in the preparation of processed food. Sodium chloride is the predominant form used, but others are also added. Look for words such as the following on your food labels:

Salt (sodium chloride)	Disodium phosphate
Monosodium glutamate (MSG)	Sodium alginate
Sodium benzoate	Sodium hydroxide
Sodium Proprionate	Sodium nitrate
Sodium sulfite	
Sodium bicarbonate (which is baking soda and also found in baking powders)	

Calcium and Phosphorus

The nutrient in current headlines is calcium. We see advertisements of bent and limping women, warnings of the risks of low intakes. Some people argue that lack of calcium, not excess sodium, is the cause of hypertension. Our bodies contain more calcium and phosphorus than any other mineral. A full 99 percent of our calcium and 80 percent of our phosphorus are bound together to form hard strong bones and teeth. The remainder circulates in the blood where they play a critical role in nerve impulses, heart and muscle contraction, blood clotting, and activation of certain enzymes. The body closely monitors calcium and phosphorus levels in the circulating blood to ensure that enough are available for these processes.

If levels drop too low, the body will step up absorption of calcium and phosphorus from the food we eat, limit loss from the kidneys, and, if necessary, take these minerals out of our bones and teeth. When circulating calcium and phosphorus are high, calcium will be replaced in the bones and teeth. They are in a constant state of flux.

An old wives' tale holds that you lose a tooth for each child. That is actually a silly thought. How would your body decide which tooth to sacrifice if more circulating calcium was needed? The calcium needs of pregnancy are high—from 800 milligrams per day for nonpregnant up to 1200 milligrams daily for pregnant women. Generally, we just become more efficient at abstracting calcium from our food and resorbing calcium in the kidneys. It is, however, an important time to make sure that we eat enough calcium-rich foods.

More frequently today we hear about the hazards of calcium deficiency as we age. Advertisements threaten us with bent and stooped backs and crooked canes if we do not down megadoses of calcium. While their claims are exaggerated, women do need to pay particular attention to calcium.

As we age, the equilibrium between the deposit and removal of calcium from the bones does change, especially in postmenopausal women whose hormones have undergone a major shift. Calcium does in fact begin to move out of the bone at a higher rate than it is replaced. The intestines become less efficient at extracting calcium from food, and the kidneys may slow a bit in their calcium-retrieving ability.

The eventual result is thinning of the bones, called osteoporosis, and an increase in fractures and back pain caused by spine compression. Approximately 1.3 million fractures occur annually among Americans over forty-five. Clearly we do not outgrow our need for calcium-rich foods like milk and other dairy products.

Lack of exercise may play as important a role in osteoporosis as does low calcium intakes. Studies in progress indicate that exercise such as bicycling or walking in moderate amounts helps maintain bone mass. The mechanism for this remains a mystery.

A number of recent studies suggest that low intakes of calcium, not high intakes of sodium, are a major factor in hypertension. There is some evidence that toxemias of pregnancy and high blood pressure may be related to calcium metabolism problems. There is not yet enough evidence to support either of these claims, though breakthrough research may provide answers in the next years.

Some concern has been expressed that the high levels of phosphorus and phosphates in our diet from meats, carbonated beverages, and certain food additives may cause calcium and bone loss. The ratio of calcium to phosphorus in the diet is critical. Some researchers are concerned that the balance is being upset by high intakes of protein and food additives. However, unless phosphorus, phosphate, or protein intakes are excessively high and simultaneously calcium intakes low, this should not present problems.

Three-fourths of the calcium in our diets comes from milk, yogurt, cheese, and other dairy products. A glass of milk, whether whole or skimmed, contains one-third of the daily requirement. Other calcium-rich foods can provide all the calcium we need. So it is probably not necessary to take a calcium supplement.

If you do choose to take a supplement, there are several major types. Bone meal is popular among those who want "natural" sources. However, it has been found to contain lead and other poisonous heavy metals. Not surprising. Our bones serve as a kind of "dumping" site to remove toxic metals from the blood.

Dolomite, a natural mineral combination of calcium carbonate and magnesium carbonate, may also contain lead. Federal safety standards have not yet been applied to these products. Until they are, several other calcium supplements are available.

Read the label to see what form of calcium is contained as this will determine the amount of calcium available (see table 2.11).

TABLE 2.11
CALCIUM SUPPLEMENTS

Type of Supplement	% Calcium
Calcium carbonate	40
Calcium lactate	13
Calcium gluconate	9
Bone meal	23–33
Dolomite	20

Many antacids contain calcium carbonate and can cost the same or less than conventional supplements.

Some manufacturers claim superior benefits from chelated calcium. A chelated mineral is one which is attached to another molecule, for example, a protein or amino acid. Chelation may or may not improve absorption. There is currently no evidence which concludes that calcium chelated with amino acids, yeast, or hydrolyzed vegetable protein is absorbed any better than calcium carbonate or other calcium salts.

From all evidence, it is important to continue to include foods in your diet which are rich sources of calcium. It is not evident that supplements are needed.

A final cautionary note: more than two-thirds of patients with a history of kidney stones had stones composed primarily of calcium salts. Exactly what causes stones to form is unclear. There is no reason to take calcium in excess of the amount recommended by the Recommended Dietary Allowances (RDA) and there may be some risks.

Trace Minerals

Trace metals or minerals are needed in microscopic amounts by our bodies. There is a very fine line between adequate amounts and toxic overdoses. These minerals are stored in the body so that borderline excessive intakes over a period of time can lead to accumulation of poisonous levels in the body. They must be present in delicate balance, as an excess of one can cause a shortage of another.

ZINC

Zinc is a trace mineral, one we need in only very small amounts. Contrary to myth, taking massive doses or eating pounds of oysters, which are high in zinc, will not increase sexual potency.

A combination of dwarfism and failure to mature sexually was first identified just over twenty years ago in Iran among people who ate an unleavened bread which caused zinc deficiency. That discovery led to folk theories about zinc and sexual potency.

While zinc deficiency does not affect willingness or ability, it has been linked to low sperm count and infertility in humans. During animal pregnancies, inadequate zinc intakes have been shown to produce birth defects and poor development of offspring.

In humans the more important role of zinc appears to be in healing wounds, fighting infections, and perhaps protecting against cancer. Zinc is critical to the proper functioning of T-lymphocytes, white blood cells which fight infections and cancer. Studies are under way to determine the role of zinc in treating severe acne. It seems to have little effect on ordinary pimples but promises to be a deterrent to pustular acne.

Lack of zinc in our diets can diminish our ability to taste and smell food and decrease our appetites.

There is disagreement about how extensive low or deficient zinc intakes may be in the United States. If they do occur it is most likely to be among people who consume very few calories for long periods of time; people who are strict vegetarians with little or no animal food products in their diet; and people who are alcoholic, have diarrheal or kidney diseases, or who are taking medications which interfere with zinc metabolism.

It is not easy to access zinc status as some dubious practitioners would have you believe. Advertisements in magazines and some questionable practitioners often offer hair analysis to determine your zinc status as well as levels of other heavy metals in your body. You send them money (the price varies from $15 to as high as $75) and a hair sample, and they send you a computer printout of "analysis" and diet/supplement recommendations.

The technology for hair analysis is still highly unreliable. Heavy metals present on the exterior of the hair, deposited from shampoos, creme rinses, and the air, will distort results. The Food and Drug Administration has brought suit against groups advertising hair analysis by mail. It asserts that hair analysis does not provide a basis for determining mineral levels or for recommending dietary supplements.

Blood analysis is more reliable but measures only circulating zinc and does not measure zinc stores. Urine analysis measures only the zinc being excreted. How much zinc is lost daily can be influenced by infections and other causes, so this too is not an accurate measure of zinc status.

Until these issues are resolved, there is no reason to take a zinc supplement. As a matter of fact, it can be quite harmful to do so without a doctor's prescription. Zinc is toxic in large amounts. We need only 15 milligrams daily. Zinc is being marketed in 50-milligram tablets—a pharmacological dose level like that used for drugs. If you take a drug equivalent you take a chance.

SELENIUM

Selenium supplements are claimed as another new miracle cure for cancer. Paradoxically, until the sixties it was considered to be a deadly toxin, causing death among cattle, horses, and sheep in Nebraska, South Dakota, Utah, and Wyoming where the soil contains a high concentration of selenium.

In the seventies it was discovered that selenium acts in concert with vitamin E to prevent a process called oxidation in the cell membranes which causes them to break down. Oxidation is caused by both natural and environmental insults. Without sufficient selenium, vitamin E cannot fend off nor repair injury to membranes.

The crucial question is does selenium prevent cancer and the jury is still out. In animal studies using very large doses, sometimes 20–30 times requirements, cancer was reduced.

Studies of blood levels of selenium in humans conclude that victims of cancer do have lower selenium levels than healthy people. However, it is not entirely clear whether the low levels help cause the cancer or whether the cancer causes the low levels. A 1983 study of blood selenium levels of 10,940 subjects revealed that those who developed cancer did have a lower selenium level before as well as after contracting cancer.

This is not a persuasive reason to rush right out for your selenium fix. Evidence that selenium might protect against cancer is incomplete and speculative. And excess intakes are highly toxic to man and animal alike.

The amount of selenium in our diets varies by the region in which we live. Those of you living in South Dakota, Wyoming, and so forth will have no difficulty getting enough selenium if you eat locally grown foods.

Selenium is not essential to plant growth. If it is around, plants will incorporate it into their cells. If it is not, they will grow without it. Therefore the level of selenium in foods is determined by which region of the country they grew in. This is very similar to iodine.

Selenium is naturally high in the soil and foods of most Midwestern states. Therefore, bread and cereal products in our diets made from grains grown in these regions will be relatively good sources of selenium.

Those of you living outside high-selenium states can get selenium from seafood and grain products like breads, rolls, pasta, and cereals. Until the RDAs specify a higher requirement or conclusive study results recommend high intakes, self-prescribed supplements probably should be avoided.

IRON

Once when my mother was tired and a bit moody and grumpy for several days, my father jokingly presented her with a bottle of Geritol to cure her "iron-poor blood." She immediately loosened up and felt better. It contains 12 percent alcohol!

Iron is the most common nutrient deficient in American diets, and iron deficiency anemia the most common deficiency disease. Because of monthly menstrual bleeding, women are more susceptive than others.

Iron enables blood cells to carry oxygen to the body's tissues, it helps bone marrow produce red blood cells, and it is a key component in a specific protein that keeps muscles working.

To ensure sufficient amounts of iron for these purposes, your body stores iron in the bone marrow, spleen, and liver. When circulating levels of iron run low, you draw iron from these reserves, just like drawing savings out of a bank. If repeated withdrawals continue without concurrent deposits, you will deplete the stores, and blood levels of iron will drop. Iron deficiency anemia occurs at this point.

Most of the iron in our bodies is in the hemoglobin, the oxygen-carrying protein which gives red blood cells their color. Any blood loss, whether from an ulcer, injury, blood donation, or menstruation, causes iron loss.

For women, monthly menstrual bleeding results in significant iron losses which must be replenished by an iron-rich diet. Women who use intrauterine devices (IUDs) for birth control lose more blood than those using other forms of contraception. Conversely, birth control pills decrease blood losses.

Pregnancy makes additional iron demands. First, blood volume swells during pregnancy, requiring more iron. The growing baby takes iron, especially during the last trimester. And large amounts of blood are lost at childbirth. For these reasons, most doctors prescribe iron supplements during and for several months after pregnancy.

If you feel tired, run down, and weak, do not self-diagnose anemia and rush out to buy iron tablets. These symptoms are common to many illnesses and conditions, including anemias caused by other deficiencies.

To determine if you are anemic, your doctor will take a blood sample and measure your hemoglobin and hematocrit. The hemoglobin measure is simply a count of the amount of hemoglobin in your blood. Normal levels range between 12 to 16 grams of hemoglobin per 100 cubic centimeters of blood. Hematocrit is a measure of how many red blood cells you have compared to other types of blood cells. That is, what percentage of blood cells are red ones. Normal values are above 38 percent. Until your hemoglobin is below 10 and your hematocrit below 31, you are not clinically iron deficient and therapeutic doses of iron are not required.

Unlike some nutrients where the body can reduce excretion when levels are low, we have no control over the amount of iron we lose. The only control is over the amount of iron absorbed from the foods we eat. On the average only 10 percent of the iron from foods is absorbed. When iron stores are low or depleted, absorption increases dramatically. However, increased absorption cannot compensate for an iron-poor diet.

The form of iron in the diet also affects absorption. Iron exists in two forms: ferrous iron with two positive charges and ferric iron with three positive charges. The ferrous form is more easily absorbed. For this reason, iron added to cereal products and supplements is usually the ferrous type.

Iron absorption can be enhanced by other nutrients. Citric acid, calcium, and vitamin C all increase absorption. So eating a vitamin C rich vegetable or fruit with a meal of iron-rich foods will increase absorption.

Iron from animal sources is more readily absorbed than iron from plant sources. For this reason, vegetarians who do not eat meats must pay special attention to iron-rich vegetables. Iron in vegetables is often in the ferric form. Eating a vitamin C rich food along with a vegetarian meal will help convert the ferric to a ferrous form and increase absorption.

Use of iron supplements should be limited to amounts at or below the Recommended Dietary Allowance (RDA). The body cannot excrete excess intakes of iron. Most iron loss occurs only through bleeding. Excess intakes are stored. Chronic overdoses can lead to toxic storage levels with damage to liver, pancreas, and heart.

IODINE

In 1920 iodine was discovered to treat goiter effectively, a condition in which the thyroid gland enlarges and causes swelling of the throat. Goiter occurs regionally in areas where the soil contains low amounts of iodine. Generally this is in areas of glacial origin or where frequent flooding occurs, leaching iodine from the soil. The goiter belt in the United States extends in a band across the top two states of the nation and around the Great Lakes area.

The most effective and inexpensive means to deliver iodine to this region was through the addition of potassium iodide to table salt. Such salt is labeled "iodized." It contains 1 part potassium iodide per 10,000 sodium chloride (table salt).

In some countries, Canada, Guatemala, Colombia, and others, where goiter continues to be a major public health problem, iodization is mandatory. In the United States it is voluntary. So both plain and iodized salts are sold.

When buying salt, it is wise to purchase iodized, even if you

do not live in the goiter belt, to ensure adequate intake of iodine. This is particularly true during pregnancy when extremely
deficient intakes can contribute to cretinism in the infant.

FLUORIDE

At the risk of being called a commie-pinko, the attributes of
fluoride do need mention. Rarely has a public health issue stirred
such debate! When incorporated into the structure of bones and
teeth, fluoride makes them stronger than hard tissues without
fluoride. The teeth are also more resistant to the cavity-causing
actions of acids produced by bacteria in the mouth as they work
on gooey, sticky sweets which adhere to our teeth. It is the single
most effective preventive measure for tooth decay.

Fluoride occurs naturally in the soil and water of some areas
of the United States. In those areas, tooth decay is significantly
lower than in areas where fluoride content of water is low. In
1945 the U.S. Public Health Service began studies to introduce
fluoride into public water supplies at the level of 1 part per
million of water (equivalent to 1 milligram per liter of water).

Since that time, in studies of over 2 million people using water
fluoridated at that level, no evidence was found of fluoride deposits in soft tissues such as the kidney or heart, no growth
abnormalities or retardation, no increase in cancer or kidney
disease, and no increase in birth defects were found.

Mottled enamel or dental fluorosis occurs only when concen-
trations exceed 2 to 8 parts per million, a level of fluoridation
not used in public water supplies. Toxicity, while possible from
overdoses of fluoride, has not occurred as a result of public water
fluoridation.

Fluoridation is a community-by-community decision, since
water supplies are locally controlled by city governments. When
a town decides to add fluoride to the water supply, the health
department first determines how much, if any, fluoride already
exists in the water. Then fluoride is added to bring the level to
between 0.7 and 1.2 parts per million.

Those who vociferously oppose fluoridation claim that it is a
compulsory intrusion of government upon their individual right
to decide about medication. Others emotionally claim a government plot to poison the populace. Never has an issue raised so
erratic a response. As a consequence, less than half of Americans
drink fluoridated water. Only seven states, Connecticut, Minnesota, Georgia, Nebraska, Ohio, South Dakota, and Kentucky,

have laws which require fluoridation of water supplies in cities of over 20,000. All other cities must individually decide what to do.

If you do not live in an area where fluoride occurs naturally in the soil and water supply and where it is not added to the municipal water supply, you can consider topical applications of fluoride and/or use of fluoridated toothpastes. Since the issue is still controversial, ask your dentist what the best route is for you.

SUPPLEMENTS

The amount of any vitamin or mineral which we need is extremely small. To demonstrate just how small, one ounce is 28.3 grams. A milligram is ¹⁄₁₀₀₀ of a gram and a microgram is ¹⁄₁₀₀₀ of a milligram. The RDA for vitamin B-12 is 6 micrograms a day. An ounce of B-12 could supply the daily needs of 4,716,667 people!

My philosophy is that if God had wanted us to take vitamin pills they would grow on trees. They don't. The only caveat to my claim is that I don't believe that God intended us to eat Twinkies, smoke cigarettes, and breathe carbon monoxide either. All of these stress the body and increase nutrient demands.

If your diet is short of important nutrients because of catch-as-catch-can and eat-on-the-run habits, the solution is not a pill. Supplements contain only those nutrients for which we specify a recommended intake level. There are other chemical components of foods whose role in our health and well-being are still unclear to us.

As the science of nutrition evolves, the importance of other nutrients and food components will be uncovered. At that time they may be added to our pills. Until then, taking a pill will provide only those components about which we have knowledge. Eating fresh and wholesome foods will give us a full range of nutrients, some of whose value is yet unknown.

Several years ago it was popular to worry about the quality of our fresh-food supply. Some warned that the soil was being depleted of nutrients and our vegetables and fruits were no longer as healthy as they once were. The solution proposed was pills.

Soil and plant scientists tell us not to worry. If the soil is low in a particular nutrient one of three results may occur. Fewer plants will grow in the area. Alternatively, the plants that grow will be smaller in size. In both cases, a carrot is a carrot is a carrot. You get fewer or smaller carrots.

Finally, there may be slight variations in the nutrients contained. But at no time will a plant be devoid of a chemical (such as carotene in carrots) which is a critical component of that plant.

One soil scientist with whom I spoke reassured me that because of the use of both chemical and organic (read: manure and compost) fertilizers, soil today is at least as rich as it was fifty years ago. So a mouthful of melon is still a better bet than a megadose of minerals.

Of far more concern to me is the continuing popularity of fluffed, puffed, processed, and packaged foods. In my opinion, they harbor hazards which cannot be fully compensated for by a pill. There is no vitamin/mineral supplement or "anticalorie" pill which can balance the potential abuse of the high-sugar, high-salt, high-fat, and low-fiber foods typical of so many American diets.

For those of you who daily eat a diet like the one in table 2.12, what is needed is a revolution in your eating patterns, not a pill. The most expensive and fanciest of vitamin/mineral supplements is no insurance policy for a diet like this.

When corporations notice that particular inputs are producing inferior products which do not hold up in appearance, do not perform to standard, and do not last, they change their inputs. If the foods listed in table 2.12 are typical of your eating habits, no patchwork or paint job will save you. It is time for a major overhaul (see table 2.13). Nor can this diet be salvaged by taking a vitamin/mineral supplement. Pills are not an insurance policy for poor eating habits.

TABLE 2.12 TYPICAL POOR DIET

Modern Menu	Calories	Fat gms	%Cal. fat	Carbo-hydrate	%Cal. carbo	Salt mgs
BREAKFAST:						
Dutch Apple Toaster Tart	210	6	26	36	69	210
Tang	90	0	0	22	100	0
Instant Coffee	tr[a]	tr[a]	tr[a]	tr[a]	tr[a]	1
Coffee Whitener	11	0.7	58	1	36	12
MID-MORNING SNACK:						
Glazed Yeast Donut	205	11	48	22	42	99
Instant Coffee	tr[a]	tr[a]	tr[a]	tr[a]	tr[a]	1
Coffee Whitener	11	0.7	58	1	tr[a]	12
LUNCH:						
Sandwich:						
White Bread, 2 slices	140	2	13	26	74	228
Mayonnaise, 1 tbsp	100	11	99	tr[a]	tr[a]	78
Am. Proc. Cheese, 1 slice	105	9	77	tr[a]	tr[a]	406
Bologna, 1 slice	85	8	85	tr[a]	tr[a]	220
Potato Chips, 10	115	8	63	10	35	200
Hawaiian Punch	130	0	0	31	95	NA
MID-AFTERNOON SNACK:						
Kool Aid	90	0	0	23	100	NA
Milk Chocolate Bar, 1 oz	145	9	56	16	44	28
DINNER:						
Frozen Breaded Fish Fillet	180	13.5	68	9	20	175
Frozen Broccoli in Cheese Sauce	70	2	26	9	52	530
Instant Mashed Potatoes	140	7	45	17	49	380
Refrigerator Biscuits	200	8	36	29	58	650
Margarine, 1 pat	35	4	100	tr[a]	tr[a]	140
Devil Food Cake/ Icing	235	8	31	40	68	402
Whole Milk	150	8	48	11	29	122
TOTAL:	2447	116	43	303	50	3894

[a] Trace amount.

TABLE 2.13 TABLE OF NEEDED NUTRIENTS

Nutrient	Food Source	Major Body Functions	Effects of Inadequacies	Effects of Excess
Carbohydrates	Cereal grains, pastas, bread, fruits, vegetables, potatoes, milk, corn, dried peas and beans, sugar, jelly, candy	Provide energy for body processes and physical activity; aid in utilization of fat and spare protein; supply 4 kcal per gram	Marasmus, weight loss, growth retardation	Weight gain and obesity
Proteins	Meat, poultry, fish, dried beans, peas, lentils, egg, cheese, milk, legumes, nuts, seeds	Provide the building material (amino acids) for growth, repair, and maintenance of every cell; regulate fluid balance between blood and cells; supply energy at 4 kcal per gram	Kwashiorkor (loss of weight and muscle mass), decreased immune response. Increased susceptibility to infection, edema	Reduced calcium retention, weight gain, and obesity
Fats	Butter, margarine, shortening, oil, lard, egg yolk, cream, salad dressing, meat and fat surrounding it, whole milk, cheese, fried foods, peanut butter	Supply energy in concentrated form; carrier of fat-soluble vitamins; supply essential fatty acids; insulate the body and promote the maintenance of normal body temperature; supply 9 kcal per gram	Flaky and scaly skin, diarrhea, poor growth, loss of hair, increased susceptibility to infection	Increased levels of triglycerides and cholesterol in the blood, accumulation of adipose tissue, weight gain, and obesity

	Sources	Function	Deficiency	Excess
Fat-soluble vitamins				
Vitamin A	Liver, carrots, sweet potatoes, dark green leafy vegetables, broccoli, winter squash, apricots, peaches, cantaloupe, milk, fish liver oil	Important component in visual process of the eye including adaptation to dark; assists in formation and maintenance of skin, mucous membranes, bones, teeth	Xerophthalmia (an eye condition leading to blindness), night blindness, permanent blindness, poor growth	Yellow pigmentation of skin, loss of appetite, vomiting
Vitamin D	Saltwater fish and their oils, fortified milk and margarine, eggs, liver, butter; can be synthesized with skin exposure to sunlight	Promotes mineralization of bones and teeth; necessary in absorption and regulation of calcium and phosphorus	Rickets (bone deformation), osteomalacia (softening of bones)	Poor growth, weight loss, vomiting, poor appetite, calcium deposition in soft tissues
Vitamin E	Seeds, fats, and polyunsaturated oils of vegetable products, whole grains	Allows vitamin A and unsaturated fatty acids to perform their specific functions; protects red blood cells from oxidation	Anemia in premature infants; no other deficiency syndrome cited for man	None reported
Vitamin K	Green leafy vegetables, liver, cabbage, peas, potatoes	Participates in formation of blood clots	Hemorrhage in newborns; in rare cases, calcium loss from bones in adults	Rarely occurs; jaundice in infants

TABLE 2.13 TABLE OF NEEDED NUTRIENTS (cont.)

Nutrient	Food Source	Major Body Functions	Effects of Inadequacies	Effects of Excess
Water-Soluble Vitamins Ascorbic Acid (Vitamin C)	Citrus fruits, strawberries, cantaloupe, cabbage, broccoli, dark green leafy vegetables, green peppers, tomatoes, potatoes	Assists in maintaining collagen (connective tissue) which gives structure to cells; promotes iron absorption; helps in wound healing	Scurvy, easy bruising, slow wound healing, fatigue, muscle ache, swollen joints, degeneration of skin, teeth, gums, and blood vessels	Increased need for vitamin C, kidney stones, interference with anticoagulant therapy and glucosuric tests
Thiamine (Vitamin B-1)	Pork, liver, oysters, cashews, whole grain and enriched breads, cereals, dried peas and beans	Assists in metabolism of carbohydrates and fats; promotes growth, good appetite, and muscle tone	Beriberi, peripheral nerve changes, edema, heart failure, loss of appetite, depression, muscle tenderness, low blood pressure	None reported
Riboflavin (Vitamin B-2)	Liver, milk and milk products, dark green leafy vegetables, whole grain breads and cereals, dried beans and peas	Assists in release of energy from proteins, fats, and carbohydrates	Chellosis (cracks at corners of the mouth), soreness of lips; redness of tongue, poor growth	None reported
Niacin	Meat, liver, fish, whole grain and enriched breads, cereals, and pastas	Key component in release of energy from fats, carbohydrates, and proteins	Pellagra, skin and gastrointestinal lesions, diarrhea, depression, anxiety	Flushing, burning and tingling around the neck and hands
Pyridoxine (Vitamin B-6)	Liver, poultry, meats, whole grain cereals, breads and pastas, bananas, nuts and seeds	Involved in metabolism of protein and amino acids; assists in red blood cell formation	Anemia, irritability, convulsions, skin lesions, peripheral nerve changes, cracks at corners of the mouth	None reported

Nutrient	Best Sources	Function	Deficiency Symptoms	Excess/Toxicity
Cobalamin (Vitamin B-12)	Meat, fish, eggs, poultry, milk and dairy products; not present in plant foods	Assists in maintenance of nerve tissue and normal blood formation	Pernicious anemia, neurological disorders	None reported
Folacin (Folic acid or folate)	Liver, dark green leafy vegetables, dried beans and peas, wheat germ	Assists in formation of red blood cells and in synthesis of genetic material	Megaloblastic anemia (enlarged red blood cells, smooth tongue, diarrhea); may cause miscarriage or small-for-date babies	None reported
Minerals				
Potassium	Bananas, orange juice, dried fruit, dried beans and peas, peanut butter, bran	Essential to fluid and electrolyte balance in cells, involved in muscle contractions	Muscle weakness, abnormal heart rhythm, kidney and lung failure	Excess in blood causes muscle paralysis and abnormal heart rate
Calcium	Milk, milk products, tofu, small canned fish with bones, dark green leafy vegetables	Needed for bone and tooth formation, blood clotting, nerve transmission for muscle contraction	Rickets, bone deformation, stunted growth in children, osteoporosis (loss of bone) with increased risk of breaks and fractures	Tiredness and drowsiness, impaired absorption of iron, zinc, magnesium, calcium
Phosphorus	Milk, milk products, meat, fish, poultry, eggs, legumes, nuts	Needed for bone and tooth formation, helps release energy from fats, carbohydrates, and proteins	Abnormal sensation of hands and feet, weakness, seizures	Distortion of calcium to phosphorus ratio, creating pseudocalcium deficiency
Zinc	Seafood, meat, eggs, liver, brewer's yeast	Part of about 100 enzymes	Poor wound healing, loss of appetite and taste, failure to grow or mature sexually	Nausea, vomiting, stomach bleeding, and abdominal pain

TABLE 2.13 TABLE OF NEEDED NUTRIENTS (cont.)

Nutrient	Food Source	Major Body Functions	Effects of Inadequacies	Effects of Excess
Selenium	Seafood, egg yolk, meat, poultry, milk, whole grain products	Prevents oxidation and breakdown of fats	None reported	None reported
Iron	Liver, kidneys, red meat, egg yolk, dried fruit (raisins, prunes), dark green leafy vegetables, whole and enriched breads, cereals, dried peas and beans	Constituent of hemoglobin in blood and myoglobin in muscles which carry oxygen to the cells	Iron deficiency anemia, fatigue, weakness, paleness, shortness of breath	Siderosis, cirrhosis of liver with toxic levels in heart and pancreas
Iodine	Saltwater fish, iodized salt, sea salt	Component of thyroid hormones; essential for normal reproduction	Goiter (enlarged thyroid on neck), cretinism and retardation in infants	None reported
Fluoride	Foods grown on soils rich in fluoride, fluoridated water, fish	Helps form strong bones, and teeth resistant to decay	Excessive tooth decay	Mottling of teeth and bones, poisonous in large doses
Magnesium	Dark green leafy vegetables, nuts, especially almonds, legumes, seeds	Aids in building proteins, helps nerves and muscles work, releases energy from muscle glycogen	Growth failure, tremors, spasms, and irregular beating of heart and muscles, leg and foot cramps	Disturbs calcium to magnesium ratio and interferes with nervous-system function

PRODUCTION COMPONENT SUMMARY

Determining the best production components would be a much easier task if there were not so much choice. John Naisbitt, in his popular book *Megatrends,* calls today the "Baskin-Robbins society." He points out that at one time there were just three flavors of ice cream: chocolate, vanilla, and strawberry. Today there are hundreds.

Since 1964, Dancer Fitzgerald Sample, a New York advertising agency, has kept track of new product introductions. In May of 1984, just one month, 226 new items were introduced. The average grocery store today contains more than 200,000 total items from which to choose.

The actual business plan to put management goals into meals and menus, follows in chapter 4. Some simple rules of thumb to help you remember the component criteria are these:

1. Contrary to many advertising claims, deficiency diseases are rare in the United States.
2. A diet which includes a wide variety of foods will protect against deficiencies. Foods contain a mixture of nutrients and can supply everything the body needs to build, repair, and operate itself.
3. Excessive intakes of calories, particularly from fats, have been tied to increased risk of obesity, kidney and heart disease. We should drastically reduce our intake of fatty foods, particularly fats which are added to our foods in cooking.
4. The foods which are listed in table 2.13 on pages 74–78 are nutrient-packed and generally low in calories. They are whole foods without excessive processing, puffing, or fluffing, and without added salt, sugar, or fat. Chapter 4 tells how to use them in quick, easy, and economical meals.
5. Each of the essential nutrients performs very specific tasks in our bodies and must be present together to do their work.
6. It is not wise to self-diagnose a condition and self-prescribe supplements to cure it without a clinical diagnosis by a doctor.
7. Excessive intakes of a vitamin or mineral, just like excessive intakes of fats and calories, can cause imbalances and health problems.

3. Trimming the Fat

"Trimming the fat" is a universal concern for corporations, governments, and businesses which wish to operate with maximum return on their investment, optimal growth rates, and assured longevity. Corporate officers monitor indicators of progress and are continually alert for ways to do business better, faster, and cheaper.

Like corporate officers, we too must look for indicators of progress toward our goals of optimal health and function and maximum life span. To monitor our own progress we must look for milestones of progress.

Body weight is the most commonly used indicator. While it doesn't tell the full story of how fit we are or how long we will live, it is certainly predictive. There is no doubt that those who are overweight suffer far more frequently from problems of high blood pressure, diabetes, atherosclerosis and heart disease, kidney stones, gout, and osteoporosis than those who are normal weight. And that those who are obese live shorter lives than those who are not.

Neither are the lives of chubby kids, overweight teenagers, portly men, and stout ladies all that jolly. They are more often filled with embarrassment with their appearance and disappointment with their inability to participate actively or comfortably in physical tasks—from simply moving gracefully to dancing to active sports or other social events.

What is a healthy weight? What weights are indicators of reduced risk of chronic disease or early death? What weights will give most social satisfaction with our appearance? Should your body weight increase with age?

STANDARDS OF WEIGHTS AND MEASURES

We have all seen tables of "ideal" or "recommended" weights. They show up in textbooks, magazines, and on the walls of our doctors' offices near the scales. What do these tables mean? Whose "ideal" are they anyway? Is this the standard for everyone to follow or just some people?

The "bible" of standard weight tables is published by the Metropolitan Life Insurance Company. Metropolitan began collecting a multitude of information on its policyholders in 1901 in order to identify risk factors to predict when death might occur.

Their purpose is to determine, based on how long they expect you to live, how much they will charge you for a life insurance policy. People who are more likely to die young must pay more since they will have a shorter period of time to pay premiums. Conversely, those people whom the company expects to live a long and healthy life and pay into the fund for long years before the policy is collected upon will be given lower policy rates.

One of the most important indicators used in predicting policyholder life expectancy is body weight. Thus "ideal" weight standards published by life insurance companies reflect the weights at which people can be expected to live the longest. A 5-foot, 10-inch man who weighs 170 pounds can expect to live longer than he would if he weighed 210 pounds. Forty pounds of pressure and weight can exert a big burden on well-being.

These tables do not predict risk of disease. They only predict life span. For example, we know that obese people more often have high blood pressure than do thin people. But we do not know the trigger point—that is, we do not know how many extra pounds of body weight will trigger high blood pressure. In fact, not all obese people will suffer from high blood pressure, even though as a group more of them will have this disorder than will a group of thin people.

We do know that for every 10 pounds you gain above normal, the risk of these diseases increases. And we do know that for each 10 extra pounds which you carry beyond the age of 35 years, your life expectancy decreases. We also know that, fortunately, this process is reversible. If you lose weight, you can decrease disease risk and add years to your life.

According to U.S. statistics in 1979, 23 million Americans, 14 percent of all males and 24 percent of all females, were more than 20 percent overweight. You can estimate how much over- or underweight you are by comparing your body weight for height and build to table 3.2.

Note that the Metropolitan tables are divided into three body types or builds. I often hear people explain extra pounds with the excuse, "I'm not really fat, I just have a large frame," which reminds me of the song lyrics, "She ain't skinny, she's just tall, that's all."

To eliminate any confusion about whether you have a small, medium, or large frame, use the following guide to determine your actual frame size before finding your "ideal" weight on the Metropolitan table.

Body Frames

Extend your arm and bend the forearm upward at a 90-degree angle. Place the thumb and the index finger of your other hand on the two prominent bones on either side of your elbow. Using a ruler or tape measure, measure the space between your fingers and compare them to table 3.1.

TABLE 3.1 MEDIUM-FRAME MEASUREMENT

Height in 1" heels	Elbow Breadth	
	Women	Men
4' 10"–4' 11"	2¼"–2½"	
5' 0"–5' 3"	2¼"–2½"	2½"–2⅞"
5' 4"–5' 7"	2⅜"–2⅝"	2⅝"–2⅞"
5' 8"–5' 11"	2⅜"–2⅝"	2¾"–3"
6' 0"–6' 3"	2½"–2¾"	2¾"–3⅛"
6' 4"		2⅞"–3¼"

Source: Courtesy of the Metropolitan Life Insurance Company.

Measurements lower than these indicate a SMALL body frame or build, while those greater than these indicate a LARGE frame.

Now locate the standard weights for your height and body frame type in table 3.2.

TABLE 3.2 1983 METROPOLITAN HEIGHT AND WEIGHT TABLES

MEN					WOMEN			
Height		Small Frame	Medium Frame	Large Frame	Height		Small Frame	Medium Frame	Large Frame
Feet	Inches				Feet	Inches			
5	2	128–134	131–141	138–150	4	10	102–111	109–121	118–131
5	3	130–136	133–143	140–153	4	11	103–113	111–123	120–134
5	4	132–138	135–145	142–156	5	0	104–115	113–126	122–137
5	5	134–140	137–148	144–160	5	1	106–118	115–129	125–140
5	6	136–142	139–151	146–164	5	2	108–121	118–132	128–143
5	7	138–145	142–154	149–168	5	3	111–124	121–135	131–147
5	8	140–148	145–157	152–172	5	4	114–127	124–138	134–151
5	9	142–151	148–160	155–176	5	5	117–130	127–141	137–155
5	10	144–154	151–163	158–180	5	6	120–133	130–144	140–159
5	11	146–157	154–166	161–184	5	7	123–136	133–147	143–163
6	0	149–160	157–170	164–188	5	8	126–139	136–150	146–167
6	1	152–164	160–174	168–192	5	9	129–142	139–153	149–170
6	2	155–168	164–178	172–197	5	10	132–145	142–156	152–173
6	3	158–172	167–182	176–202	5	11	135–148	145–159	155–176
6	4	162–176	171–187	181–207	6	0	138–151	148–162	158–179

Weights at ages 25–59 based on lowest mortality. Weight in pounds according to frame (in indoor clothing weighing 5 lbs, shoes with 1-in. heels).

Weights at ages 25–59 based on lowest mortality. Weight in pounds according to frame (in indoor clothing weighing 3 lbs, shoes with 1-in. heels).

Source: Courtesy of the Metropolitan Life Insurance Company. Basic data from 1979 *Build Study*, Society of Actuaries and Association of Life Insurance Medical Directors of America, 1980.

Tables 3.1 and 3.2 apply to adults. The most current reference for standard heights and weights for children comes from the Medical College of Wisconsin (see chart).

FIT OR FAT?

"Ideal" weight tables compare weight to height and body build. They do not indicate what percentage of that body weight is bone, or muscle, or fat. It is possible to be 145 pounds and fat or 145 pounds and fit. It all depends on the percentage of body weight which is fat.

It is also possible to weigh considerably more than the tables recommend and still be fit. Football players, heavyweight wrestlers, and weight lifters often weigh more than is suggested by

Average Height and Weight for Children

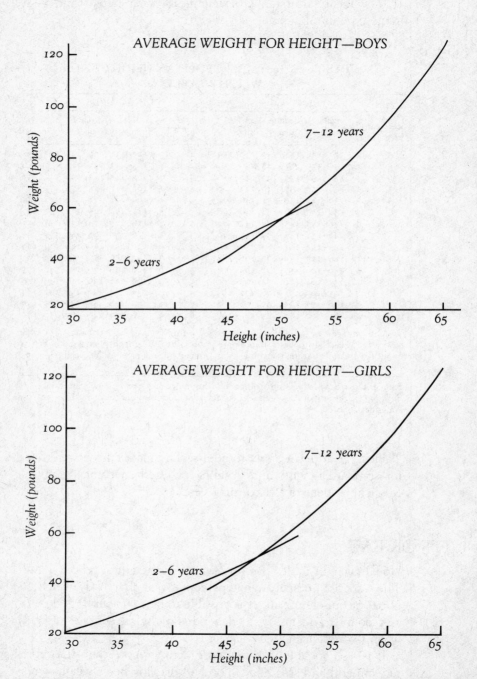

AVERAGE WEIGHT FOR HEIGHT—BOYS

AVERAGE WEIGHT FOR HEIGHT—GIRLS

Source: Prepared by A. Rimm, Ph.D., A. Hartz, M.D., Ph.D., et al., using data from National Center for Health Statistics, Medical College of Wisconsin, 1984.

the tables. Their bodies are heavily muscled, and muscle is denser and weighs more than fat. Likewise, it is possible to weigh less than the standards and be unfit, if you have very little muscle tissue.

A highly trained female athlete carries only 10–20 percent of her weight as body fat. The rest is taut muscles and strong bones. Grete Waitz, seven times female winner of the New York City Marathon, is approximately 9 percent body fat. Joan Benoit, winner of the 1984 Olympic women's marathon is 6–7 percent fat. The majority of the rest of us are 25–35 percent fat, an excess of about 10 percent more than the 20–25 percent which is healthy and attractive.

Men should aim for 15–20 percent or less body fat. Again, highly trained athletes are considerably less fat than this. Alberto Salazar, winner of the 1980 New York men's marathon, is 4.6 percent.

Measures to Determine Body Fat

The most accurate method to determine the real amount of your weight which is fat would be to analyze your cadaver. Clearly this has its limitations! Therefore, we must rely on indirect methods of estimating total body fat. Several complicated and expensive techniques are used in laboratories.

X-rays and sonograms are used to outline the shadow of fat surrounding organs and to measure how dense fat deposits are. This is not an extremely accurate estimate of total fat.

Radioactive tracer dyes, which disperse through the water in the body, can be injected into the body and then measured. Since fat cells contain less water than other cells, a calculation can be made to estimate percentage body fat.

Another expensive technique, called potassium scintillation, measures the amount of naturally occurring potassium. Less potassium is present in fat tissues than in muscle and bone. High proportional weight to low potassium counts indicates a high percentage of weight as fat. None of these methods are widely used and all are very expensive.

Densitometry

A more commonly used and safe method of determining percentage body weight as fat, is hydrostatic (underwater) weigh-

ing. This method is based on a very simple principle: fat floats!
You have observed this when you make salad dressing at home.
The oil (a liquid fat) floats to the top of the bottle while the
water and vinegar go to the bottom.

Fat tissue is less dense than either muscle or bone, called lean
tissues. It will float. Thus a person weighing 145 pounds with a
great deal of that weight as fat will float, while a trained wrestler
weighing the same but with more muscle and lean tissue will
sink.

In hydrostatic weighing, a comparison is made of your weight
in air to your weight when completely submerged in water. Cor-
rections are made for the amount of air in the lungs and gastroin-
testinal tract, since these will make you float. A person with a
low percentage of fat will weigh more underwater than a person
of similar weight who has more fat. The fat person will float—
like a cork.

From these measurements, a calculation is made to estimate
percentage of body fat. The technique is accurate, not excessively expensive, but also not portable. Only a few underwater
labs exist nationally. They are generally used in research and
for training athletes. Most are not yet available to the
public.

Pinch Test

A more widely available technique is the use of skinfold calipers
to measure the amount of fat under the skin. Our bodies store
fat just under the skin surface as insulation against severe
changes in temperature and damage to the body from puncture,
pressure, or impact. It protects us just like a combination electric
blanket and ice hockey players' padding.

About 50 percent of our fat is stored subcutaneously, under
the skin. It follows that the thicker the skinfold (a fold of skin
and fat, but not the underlying muscle) the greater the amount
of fat a person is carrying. To measure this subcutaneous layer,
specially designed calipers (pincers) are used which measure the
thickness of representative sites throughout the body. These
measurements are then put into a mathematical equation to
estimate the body's density and percent fat.

Skinfold calipers are inexpensive, portable, and appropriate
for use in both laboratory and field settings when used by experienced and skilled individuals. They are commonly used by
schools, athletic teams, YM/YWCAs, and related health cen-

ters. Pediatricians and other doctors use them for a handy and quick estimate of percentage of body fat.

If you do not have access to these more sophisticated estimates of body fatness, two other standby tests exist. While not as accurate as any of the above tests, they are telling enough to be used by doctors and nutritionists.

The first is a do-it-yourself pinch test. You might remember that your pediatrician pinched your cheeks and also just above and behind your elbows and around your midriff just below your ribs. By doing so he or she could tell how fat you were. Generally, if you can pinch an inch, you have excess body fat. This rule of thumb applies to adults too.

Finally, there is the old standby "Mirror, Mirror on the Wall" test. Disrobe and stand in front of a full-length mirror. Now cast a critical eye over your body—front, back, and side views. Are there sags? bags? bulges? irregular curves? lack of muscle definition? A fit body is firm with visible muscle contours. Really look and tell the truth!

FAT AND FORTY

Notice that the table of "ideal" weights makes no reference to age. There is no assumption that as we age we will or should gain weight. Yet that is what we commonly do. A professor of mine at Berkeley contends that you can guess a person's age by his or her weight.

Unfortunately, her theory has been confirmed by studies. The national Health and Nutrition Examination Survey, conducted every three years by the federal government, found that at age 18 a female of 5 feet, 4 inches, will weigh approximately 120 pounds, and by age 40 she will weigh 148 pounds.

Two factors are at play. First, changes in body composition do occur as we age. The amount of muscle tissue and the mass of our bones diminish slightly as we age. To compensate, there is a slight increase in body fat and thus a slight rise in body weight.

Second, our metabolism does slow slightly as we age. In part this is due to the decrease in active muscle tissue and in part due to changes in our functioning organs and tissues.

These changes are not inevitable nor irreversible. Ten years ago when a movie star reached the age of 35 she was considered a has-been. Today (1985) among our most sizzling and sexy stars are Dolly Parton at 39, Tina Turner at 43, Jane Fonda at 47,

Linda Evans at 43, Joan Collins at 49, Rita Moreno at 53, and Diana Ross at 41.

Ten years ago a model's career was over at 22. Today, along with the above stars, *Vogue, Harper's Bazaar*, and other high-fashion magazines carry cover photos of models well into their forties. Frequent cover articles hail the glories of beauty into the midyears.

Fat and forty is fast becoming unfashionable. Concern with physical fitness has increased among those over forty just as it has among all ages. More aging citizens are spending their spare time and interest in physical activities and exercise, with a resulting increase in physical fitness and a decrease or stabilization of weight. They are reversing the old pattern of debility and dependence that once accompanied aging.

We can look forty before we are, if we are fat. Aging and disuse are virtually indistinguishable, physiologically. The adage "Use it or lose it" is true. Unused muscles will deteriorate and be replaced with flab and fat. We can begin to sag and bag well before our years. However, if we remain active and participate faithfully in aerobic, stretching, and flexing exercises, we can avoid much of the infiltration of fat and retain our youthful stride and bounce.

MIRROR, MIRROR

Appearance is probably the most important of social factors influencing our success, personally and professionally. It is certainly the most powerful creator of first impressions.

Studies show that people who are overweight earn less income than thin people and do not enjoy the same rate of job advancement or salary increases as those who are normal weight. When questioned, employers reported that they thought that overweight people were slow and lacked self-confidence. Furthermore, they thought that anyone who could not control his or her weight could not control budgets, personnel, and production projects.

A survey conducted by Robert Half International Inc., an executive-recruitment agency, concluded that among 180 jobs studied, salaries for executives who regularly participated in one or more sports—swimming, running, tennis, or handball—earned an average of $3,120 more per year than executives who did not participate regularly in physical activities.

There is clearly a prejudice against overweight. But has this always been so? The lithe look idolized by Americans today is a recent obsession. At one time, obesity was a mark of status, suggesting that the person did not have to perform ordinary manual labor to earn a living. Paintings by the old masters, portraying life among the elite, hailed the heavy. What we would describe as fat was favorable and fashionable to Titian, Rubens, and their peers. In many cultures this is still the value.

In America, the struggle to cross the continent and settle the Western badlands took great physical endurance and strength, leaving very little fat or fluff on those who survived the crossing. Yet the paintings which hung in gold rush and boom town bars were of zaftig, that is, voluptuous, women and corpulent, dapper men. Hardship was associated with leanness; success with rotund weight.

The "ideal" figure for men has changed less over the decades than has the ideal for women. We still associate overweight in men with success, in part because overweight tends to occur at middle age when a man has generally established his career. We expect the successful businessman to have a three-martini lunch and client dinners at fancy restaurants. We excuse the extra weight this produces as the price and mark of achievement.

As we have become more affluent as a society, American men have gained weight. Statistics on military service recruits show that men 5 feet, 10 inches and aged 30–34 who entered the Union Army in 1863 weighed about 147 pounds on average. In 1960–62 the average weight of men in that same height and age category was 170 pounds, a 33-pound increase. There are indications from subsequent government reports that American men have continued to gain girth.

Curiously, the "ideal" figure for men tends to follow or reflect what is happening with their weights rather than to set trends which they must follow. Unless a man becomes extremely obese, he seldom worries about his weight, seldom feels any loss of self-esteem, and does not fear the loss of respect of others.

Only in the last five years has any attention been given to a leaner man. Burt Reynolds in his landmark centerfold for *Playgirl* magazine was beguilingly plump. Today's foldouts are linear, lean, and sinewy.

A similar change has taken place in perceptions of the ideal feminine figure. Gone are the billowy, buxom Gibson girls.

Gone are Marilyn Monroe, Jayne Mansfield, and Jane Russell with their wide hips, plushy pursed lips, and ample bosoms. And gone are the days when the overweight woman is looked upon as either rich or successful. When Babe Paley, wife of CBS executive William Paley, announced in the sixties that a woman could never be too thin or too rich, she heralded an era that was to spawn the 95-pound Twiggy, Gloria Vanderbilt, and other little-boy look-alikes.

The early seventies, with emphasis on career competence, competition, and entry into the male-dominated business world, continued the popularity of unisex figures for women. Some of this emphasis has continued, although it has softened as we now have male-style underwear in pastels with lace offered for purchase by women.

Women are building their bodies—not to look like men but rather to express their strength and physicality as females. Actresses who once published weighty memoirs are now publishing weight-lifting guides.

Our grandmothers, women who crossed the Plains for California, swam the Rio for Texas, survived the camps in Germany, or harvested the crops in the South, were no frail fledglings. They were women of strength and endurance. And they were feminine.

The new woman has that same physical quality. She is healthy, athletic, outdoorsy, exercised, limber, and at the same time not afraid of frail frills, lilting lace, or silk stockings.

Clothing sizes, as well as clothing styles, change to reflect changes in our bodies. The Wolf Form Company in New York City builds the majority of torso dummy dress forms used by clothing designers and manufacturers in the United States and Europe. Each form is individually made and meets measurements supplied by the manufacturer. The company says that American women have changed over the past fifty years. Their hips are slightly larger, their breasts smaller and lower, and they are more athletic than before.

There are no national standards nor any national center for collecting information on how our bodies are changing. However, large clothing retailers, like Sears, Roebuck, J. C. Penney, Macy's, and Montgomery Ward, do monitor changes. In 1978, Sears announced revisions in its size 10 measurements to enlarge the hips and waist and decrease the size of the bust. (See table 3.3.)

TABLE 3.3 MEASUREMENTS OF
AVERAGE AMERICAN WOMAN
(SIZE 10)

Height	5 ft 4 in.
Weight	130 lb
Bust	37 in.
Waist	29 in.
Hips	39 in.
Thighs	23 in.
Calves	14 in.

IS A CALORIE ALWAYS A CALORIE?

In the face of our desire to be perfect 10s, why would our bodies defeat us by storing fat? Surely something is wrong!

Until a year or so ago, scientists and obesity researchers contended that a calorie was a calorie, no matter what its source, and that an excess of 3500 calories produced a pound of body fat. Pure and simple mathematics!

Researchers today are more skeptical. One simple truth remains: if you eat or drink more calories than your body needs, it will store the excess as fat. However, what constitutes "excess" may not be as straightforward and simple as was once believed.

Evidence is growing that a calorie is not always a calorie. Recall that a calorie is a measure of energy—specifically the amount of energy required to raise the temperature of 1 gram of water 1 degree centigrade. When viewed in this way, it does not matter whether a single calorie is from fat, sugar, or protein. Water doesn't care what the source of energy is.

Apparently our bodies do care. Use of calories by the body is not a simple physical transfer of heat as it is when calories are burned to heat water. It is a complex set of chemical reactions involving many nutrients, enzymes, metabolites, and intermediary steps where a number of biochemical decisions can be made by the body about what to do with the calories.

The source of calories in our diets, the size of meals, the time of day at which they are eaten, and the frequency with which we eat, all influence whether and to what degree we store fat cells. And some people are more efficient in using and storing calories than others.

Fattening Foods

One rule that seems to be true about food is that it is the only place in life where you can eat your cake and have it too. A moment on the lips, forever on the hips!

It is conventional wisdom that some foods are just more fattening than others—sadly, many times the foods which we love best. Even looking at pictures or recipes of these foods seems to make us fat.

But is this really so? Will a 500-calorie slice of chocolate mousse fudge cake make us fatter than a 500-calorie meal of salad, fish, potato, and a vegetable?

It just might. When we eat a meal high in sugar or a slice of cake, our blood sugar rises sharply. Simple sugars are absorbed fairly rapidly from the stomach into the bloodstream. Our body then releases insulin, a hormone which regulates the level of sugar and fat in the blood and body cells. Insulin moves the sugar from the bloodstream into the body cells. Muscle cells will use the sugar for immediate energy or store unused amounts, in small quantities, as glycogen. Fat cells convert the sugar to fat and store it until it is needed for energy.

Most of the calories in a slice of chocolate mousse fudge cake will be in the form of sugar or fat, relatively pure calories. If the body does not need these calories for immediate energy, they will be stored.

A mixed meal of foods containing protein, fats, complex and simple carbohydrates takes longer to digest and metabolize. The protein will be used to build and repair body tissues rather than to provide calories. The complex carbohydrates will be broken down to release the simple sugars which compose them. The fats will be sent to storage if they are not needed for energy. This all takes time.

Only the simple sugar portion of the meal will be absorbed quickly to induce an immediate insulin response. The other components—protein, fat, and complex carbohydrate—will take perhaps 2–3 hours to reach the bloodstream, producing a slow and sustained level of sugar in the blood.

The result is that energy is readily available as it is needed and you do not feel hungry. A mixed meal eliminates peaks and valleys of energy and you will be less likely to return to the cupboard for another piece of cake in an hour.

The protein will be used for purposes other than energy. More energy will be required to digest and metabolize these more complex nutrients and fewer of the 500 calories will be stored as fat. The mixed meal will also give you a good dose of vitamins and minerals which do not alter your appetite but do improve your intake of essential nutrients.

Eats All Day

One of the people you may dislike most in life is the skinny guy who seems to eat all day without gaining a pound. Studies indicate that eating small, frequent meals may do more to control weight than eating the same number of calories at one or two large meals.

Insulin may again be involved. Large meals trigger release of insulin which in turn increases fat storage. Small meals tend to release insulin in smaller, more sustained amounts, creating an even insulin and blood sugar level and less fat storage. Small, frequent meals ensure a constant source of readily available energy, without excess for storage.

Dieters' Dinner

Skipping breakfast and dieting at lunch are a popular panacea which unfortunately does not work. There are two reasons for this.

First, a dieter who arrives at the dinner table ravenously hungry is far more likely to eat everything which doesn't move and also to eat seconds, than a dieter who arrives at the table only mildly hungry. That one meal eaten when you feel starved can contain more calories than several smaller meals.

Second, even if you did not overeat, you would lose less weight if all your calories were eaten at night than if they are spread throughout the day or eaten early in the day. Studies at the National Institutes of Health showed that women who ate a fixed number of calories lost more weight when they ate all their food in the morning than when they ate the same amount in the evening.

A University of Minnesota study gave a single test meal of 2000 calories. If eaten in the morning, subjects actually lost weight. If eaten at dinnertime, subjects either lost less weight or gained weight.

The explanation for this seems to be that food eaten at night is not burned for energy, since you are not exercising. It is stored as fat while you sleep. Eating should be followed by activity in order to get the calorie-burning mechanisms going. The best way to achieve this is to eat early in the day when you are active.

"Breakfast like a king, lunch like a prince, and dine like a pauper" may be excellent advice for the weight conscious.

No Matter What I Eat, It Turns to Fat

The basic total number of fat cells in our body is established in childhood. Fat babies are more prone to become fat teenagers and fat adults than are average-weight infants. Once the fat cells are laid down, they never disappear. They shrink when weight is lost and fill with fat when weight is gained. They may slightly increase in number, but they do not change significantly.

The typical lean person has about 27 trillion fat cells. A typical obese person has 77 trillion fat cells. When their fat cells are filled, obese people have both more fat cells and fatter fat cells than lean people.

Fat people do not necessarily eat more than thin or normal-weight people. Studies indicate they may eat about the same or slightly less food. Still, they do eat more calories than they need for their level of body activity. Typically, obese people are far less active than normal-weight people.

This is particularly true of obese children. Studies of children playing various group games in a schoolyard reveal that overweight children move less often and less quickly than normal and thin children. They burn fewer calories because they are less active.

The same thing happens as we age. We tend to become less active. When we graduate from school and enter the work force or marry and begin to raise a family, we become more sedentary. We devote less time to sports activities which were part of our school day. We may have walked to school but now drive to work and to do errands. We no longer dance until dawn but are up at dawn, into our cars, and on our way to work where most of us will sit most of the day. When we retire, we may reduce our activity level even further.

Our metabolic rate, that is the rate at which we burn calories for energy, is not a fixed rate. When we exercise, our metabolic rate speeds up. When we sleep, sit, or move slowly, it slows down.

Some of us may be slightly more efficient in the use of calories than others. For efficient energy users, less than 3500 calories may produce a pound of weight. Even though the metabolic burners may burn slower for some people than for others, activity will still push up the rate of calorie burning.

Whether efficient or not, the rule still holds that to lose weight, you must burn more calories than you eat. If you are someone who is an inefficient calorie burner, someone with "slow metabolism" as it is commonly called, you can increase your metabolic rate by increasing activity. You should not simply give up and excuse excess flab as "my metabolism."

Curiously, going on a diet to decrease calorie intake produces less rapid and less stable weight loss than pushing up your metabolic rate by increased activity.

If you think about it, you know this from your own experience. How many times have you gone on an 800–1000 calorie diet, lost 10 pounds, only to gain it back in two weeks?

Our bodies compensate for reduced calorie intake by becoming more efficient in calorie use. It is as if someone turned the thermostat down because there was a fuel shortage. Our bodies make adjustments to conserve energy when there is less energy available.

When we go off the diet, our body temporarily remains in the efficiency mode. It replaces the fat which was burned during the shortage and the nutrients which were depleted. We balloon back to our previous weight and blame ourselves for failing to stick to the diet.

Very-low-calorie diets are contrary to our body's survival instinct. They work against rather than with our bodies. If such diets did work, there would be no market for the "diet of the month"—the burgeoning bookshelves and newsstands of fad diets. What does seem to work is a well-balanced diet, containing a wide variety of foods which provide all the essential nutrients and fiber which your body needs. AND EXERCISE.

The Anticalorie

Evidence is rapidly accumulating that the body's thermostat can be reset and calorie burning speeded by exercise (see table 3.4). Benefits occur not only during the exercise period when calories are burned to support the activity, but the rate of burn remains elevated for a period after exercise ceases. Studies indicate that the body burns up to 20 percent more calories in the two- to four-hour period following a half-hour exercise period than it would burn if no exercise occurred.

Moderate exercise also reduces appetite. It is not clear how this mechanism works. When we exercise extensively, our appetities increase and we eat to compensate for the calories burned. However, when we exercise only a moderate amount, ½ to 1 hour, appetites are suppressed. Elevated body temperature following exercise may be the cause. It is not clear.

In the unexercised, sedentary body, this appetite-regulating mechanism fails. Food intake is not adjusted to match energy expenditure. Farmers use this knowledge to fatten hogs, cattle, and chickens for market. They cage them to restrict their activity. The animals' appetite-regulating mechanisms fail and they overeat, becoming fat for market.

My father's theory is that the best exercise for dieters is pushing themselves away from the table. While that is certainly advisable and does spare you from seconds, it does not burn many calories.

An overweight patient of mine declared that exercise was an unreasonable means of losing weight. She pointed out that it would take 11⅙ hours of walking, 5½ hours of swimming, or 7½ hours of bicycling to lose just 1 pound of fat. She said that she was unwilling to face such an ordeal.

She began to listen when I reassured her that exercise will produce that result even when divided into several days. If she were to bicycle vigorously for ½ hour daily, she could lose 1 pound in a week and up to 26 pounds of fat in a year. This sounded more reasonable to her.

Further, she rapidly changed her snacking patterns when she learned how much exercise she would have to perform in order to burn off the calories in her favorite snacks. Since she hated to exercise, she began eating apples so that she had to run only 5 minutes rather than to run the 22 minutes needed to burn off the calories in a milk shake.

Surprisingly, the types of activities in which we are engaged for the majority of our time do not use a lot of calories. Table 3.5 shows average calories spent for various activities. Notice that for activities like typing, driving, reading, and so forth, we burn only about 1⅓ calories per hour for each kilogram (about 2.2 pounds) that we weigh. Thus a 110-pound woman would burn less than 600 calories for a full day of very light activity.

TABLE 3.4 MINUTES OF ACTIVITY REQUIRED TO BURN CALORIES

Food	Calories	Walk	Bi-cycle	Swim	Run	Sit Relaxed
Carrot, raw	42	8	5	4	2	32
Peach, medium	46	9	6	4	2	35
Orange, medium	68	13	8	6	4	52
Potato chips, 10	108	21	13	10	6	83
Doughnut, 1	151	29	18	13	8	116
Ice cream, ⅙ qt	193	37	24	17	10	148

Source: Frank Konishi, "Food Energy Equivalents of Various Activities," Copyright the American Dietetic Association. Reprinted with permission, *Journal of the American Dietetic Association*, Vol. 46: 186, 1965.

Using table 3.5, you can estimate the number of calories you burn in a day. First record the number of hours spent in each type of activity. Then multiply each total time by your weight in kilograms (your weight divided by 2.2 will give your weight in kilograms). Next multiply by the calories for that type of activity. For example, see table 3.6 for a 110-pound (50 kilograms) woman's day.

TABLE 3.5 ENERGY REQUIRED BY VARIOUS ACTIVITIES

Activity	Men (kcal/body wt in kg/hour) [a]	Women (kcal/body wt in kg/hour) [a]
Sleep and reclining	1.1	1.0
Very light activity		
Seated and standing activities, painting, auto and truck driving, typing, sewing	1.5	1.3
Light		
Walking (2.5–3 mph), carpentry, restaurant trades, washing clothes, golf, volleyball	2.9	2.6
Moderate		
Walking (3.5–4 mph), weeding, hoeing, scrubbing floors, cycling, tennis, dancing	4.3	4.1
Heavy		
Walking with load up hill, tree cutting, working with pick and shovel, swimming, climbing, football	8.4	8.0

[a] These are average figures. Variation occurs between individuals based on age, intensity of exercise, and body size.

Source: Adapted from "Recommended Dietary Allowances," 1980.

TABLE 3.6 CALORIES BURNED IN A DAY

Activity	Hr	Kg	Kcal
Sleep	8.0 x 50 x 1.0	=	400
Very light	9.0 x 50 x 1.3	=	585
Light	4.5 x 50 x 2.6	=	585
Moderate	1.5 x 50 x 4.1	=	307
Heavy	1.0 x 50 x 8.0	=	400
			2277 total calories used

You do not have to become a marathon runner in order to lose weight and increase your fitness level. Any exercise which increases heart rate to above 120–130 beats per minute (the rate for 25–35 years old) will increase the calorie burning rate. Exercise at this rate for 200 minutes per week (about 30 minutes daily) can burn an extra 2000 calories.

Two types of exercise are needed: those to improve your heart function and increase circulation and breathing such as jogging or swimming. And those to improve strength, agility, flexibility, coordination and muscle tone such as calisthenics or gymnastics.

Choose an exercise which you enjoy rather than one which you dislike so that the exercise itself will be a reward. Find activities which are convenient and all-weather so that you will have no excuses not to do them. I am not talking about finger exercises or fork lifting to the mouth!

You do not have to do the same exercise every day. You could walk to work or the store on Monday. Attend a calisthenics class on Tuesday. Play tennis on Wednesday. Jog on Thursday.

You can also find ways to increase calorie burning while going about your normal daily activities. If you need to go ten blocks away on an errand, walk them rather than drive or ride. If you want to go up 3–4 floors, walk rather than ride the elevator. And definitely walk down anything less than 7–8 floors.

Put your motorized lawn mower in storage and sharpen up the man-powered model. Take a 20-minute brisk walk or a brief bicycle ride after dinner instead of plopping yourself in front of the television with a bag of goodies to nibble during the evening sitcoms.

My husband is a long-distance runner who doesn't need a list of extra little calorie burning exercises. So he suggests that I do the dishes rather than he to ensure that I keep in shape! It always helps to have a family who supports you in your efforts to keep trim.

Fitness is not a sometimes proposition. Unfortunately, it is not like spring cleaning, done once a year. It is a full-time maintenance job. Calories can be stockpiled for future needs. The benefits of exercise cannot. You have to renew them daily.

We are not only what we eat, we are also what our muscles make us: weak or strong, fat or fit, energetic or lethargic. The benefits of exercise far exceed their ability to burn calories. People who exercise regularly have an enhanced sense of well-being and a positive outlook on life. They experience less tension, strain, and stress. Their mental and physical performance is improved, as is their endurance, stamina, flexibility, and grace. They suffer far less frequently from cardiovascular diseases such as stroke and heart attack. And even as they age, if they exercise regularly, their bodies will retain strength, agility, and a youthful appearance and motion.

4. Home, Inc., Business Plan

It is now time to put together the plan—the meals and menus which will meet the multiple nutrition and life-style needs of the family and keep both budget and bulges to a minimum.

It is critical to have a plan. Decisions made without one can result in chaos: lost time, squandered money and energy, inadequate nutrient intake, excessive calories, and/or meals which are unappealing and unappetizing.

No successful business, whether owner-operated or a multinational conglomerate, operates without a business plan or strategy, a master guide for decision making. These plans do not appear by some miracle, nor are they delivered by an oracle of God or from top management down to company employees. They evolve over time and are continually in the process of adjustment and adaptation to changing circumstances.

A business plan is a blueprint for decisions and action. It is a design for a specific course of action to make sure that the right things happen, on schedule and within fiscal constraints. Plans leave little to happenstance or accident.

As managers of family nutrition and health, it is our responsibility to ensure that family food habits do not occur haphazardly. That requires planning. Crisis solutions almost always yield long-term results which are poorer, more costly, and less efficient than planned interventions.

MENUS TO END MUDDLING THROUGH

The foundation of all health is a balanced diet which provides all the protein, fat, carbohydrates, vitamins, and minerals which our bodies need to build, repair, and replace tissues and to function normally and actively.

Balance means that the diet has just enough of all the essential elements and not too much of anything. It results from eating a wide variety of wholesome foods.

From the previous chapter you will recall that some foods are better sources of nutrients than others. Some foods, calorie for calorie, provide little nutrition and negative health consequences as well. If we select foods carefully, we can eat wholesome, healthful meals which are low-calorie, low-cost, and quick.

Recall that everyone in the family needs the same nutrients, just in different amounts. You do not need to become a slave to the stove, preparing a separate meal for each family member. Altering portion sizes is all that is required, including for dieters.

It is also true that we regularly eat about the same types of food at about the same time of day. Some people eat three snacks and only one main meal. Some eat two meals and a snack. Most people can be divided into one of three groups who eat as follows:

Pattern I: 3 meals and 1 snack
Pattern II: 3 meals and 2 snacks
Pattern III: 2 meals and 2 snacks

To get you started planning menus, I have designed three menu patterns which follow these typical eating patterns. Select the pattern which is most like how you and your family members currently eat. Then follow through the planning process to see how you can control calories, cost, and time while meeting everyone's nutritional needs from the same menu.

Two variations for each pattern will be shown: one provides between 1600 and 1800 calories daily and the other provides approximately 2200 to 2400 calories.

Calorie needs are an individual matter, determined by age, sex, body size, and level of activity. Table 4.1 lists the average energy (calories) needed by each family member. The lowest values in the range are for persons who are inactive. The highest values are for people who engage in heavy physical labor and extensive physical exercise.

TABLE 4.1 RECOMMENDED ENERGY INTAKES BY MEAN HEIGHTS AND WEIGHTS

Category	Age (yr)	Weight (lb)	Height (in.)	Energy Needs in Kcal	
				Average	Range
Infants	0–½	13	24		95–145
	½–1	20	28		80–135
Children	1–3	29	35	1300	900–1800
	4–6	44	44	1700	1300–2300
	7–10	62	52	2400	1650–3300
Males	11–14	99	62	2700	2000–3700
	15–18	145	69	2800	2100–3900
	19–22	154	70	2900	2500–3300
	23–50	154	70	2700	2300–3100
	51–75	154	70	2400	2000–2800
	76 +	154	70	2050	1650–2450
Females	11–14	101	62	2200	1500–3000
	15–18	120	64	2100	1200–3000
	19–22	120	64	2100	1700–2500
	23–50	120	64	2000	1600–2400
	51–75	120	64	1800	1400–2200
	76 +	120	64	1600	1200–2000
Pregnancy				+ 300	
Lactation				+ 500	

Source: Adapted from "Recommended Dietary Allowances," 1980.

Notice from the above chart that daily meal plans which provide either 1600–1800 calories or 2200–2400 calories will meet the needs of most individuals.

By simply changing the number of foods selected or the serving size, the calories in each pattern can be increased or decreased to meet the needs of all your family members.

For example, a 10-year-old boy will need around 2200–2400 calories as will his father who has a job sitting behind a desk. A five-year-old boy and his mother probably need about the same 1600–1800 calories. An active teenager will need more calories than an inactive one, so you can increase serving sizes to provide more calories.

If you are dieting, you may want to lower calorie level slightly by decreasing serving sizes. However, recall from chapter 3 that increasing calorie output through exercise is a more effective way to lose pounds and inches.

HOW IT WORKS

If you have ever been to a Chinese restaurant for dinner, you will be an expert at this menu system. It is as easy as selecting foods from a menu written in a language you do not read. You simply pick one item from column a, two from column b, and so forth. And you pray that what you ordered was not bird's nest soup or 100-year-old eggs!

Meals are made from foods which can be grouped according to the nutrients they provide. For example, all the dairy products and tofu are excellent sources of calcium, phosphorus, and protein. All the treats like candy and cookies are full of fat, sugar, calories, and generally cost more than they return on your food budget!

To form the columns for our Chinese restaurant menu system, the foods have been grouped according to the dominant nutrients which they provide. Milk products and tofu are in the dairy foods group. Cookies and candies are in the treats group.

The foods in each group have a serving or portion size listed. These serving sizes contain approximately the same number of calories. This will allow you to interchange foods within the group. So if you feel like having one small pear for lunch instead of twelve grapes, they will have about the same number of calories.

Portion control is essential to good management. Restaurant chefs do not randomly place food on a plate. They use specific utensils to control portion size. Their purpose is to ensure that they do not run short of food for the number of guests expected and to control cost.

Portion control at home can be a means of controlling calories as well as cost. It is simple arithmetic. A half cup serving of ice cream has half the number of calories as a full cup and costs half as much. Pay strict attention to serving sizes, especially for dieters. Calories and costs can edge up by the teaspoon and the ounce to give you an uncontrolled waistline and wallet.

Let's get started. First you will see how the foods are grouped. There are seven groups:

Dairy foods   Carbohydrates
Fruits   Fats and oils
Vegetables   Treats
Protein foods

Each group has a short explanation of the important nutrients contained and the average calories in the serving sizes listed.

Next we will look at the three meal patterns to see how the food groups are used to plan meals and snacks.

Then you will find sample menu ideas and tips for putting a meal in a bag, grabbing it on the run, cooking it right to cut calories, and quick, easy meals from bare cupboards.

Dairy Foods

These foods are rich in calcium, protein, riboflavin, vitamins A and D.

The calories in dairy foods come predominantly from the butter fat contained. Therefore, as the fat content increases, the calories increase. To provide the same number of calories in each serving, the serving size of higher fat products must decrease (see table 4.2). For example, compare the serving size of skim to that of whole milk. Also, the more fat a dairy product contains, the more expensive it is. This is good news. Low-fat, low-calorie in this groups means low-cost.

TABLE 4.2 DAIRY FOODS GROUP
(Approximately 100 Calories)

1½ cups skim milk
1 cup low-fat milk
¾ cup whole milk
1 cup low-fat buttermilk
1 cup low-fat plain yogurt
1½ slices (1½ oz) cheese

Fruits

Nearly all the vitamin C in our diets comes from this group. As we discussed in chapter 2, our bodies do not store vitamin C. So it is important to include a vitamin C rich food from this group in our diets every day (see table 4.3).

Fruits also contain vitamin A, other vitamins, and minerals, simple fruit sugars, and fiber. They are the only "sweets" which we need in our diets and can provide major savings if substituted for sugar-filled snack foods. (See page 170.)

TABLE 4.3 FRUIT GROUP
(Approximately 50 Calories)

1 small apple, orange,[a] pear	1 medium peach, fig, tangerine[a]
2 medium plums, apricots, prunes, dates	1/3 cup cranberry, apple, pineapple juice
1/4 cup prune juice, grape juice, apricot nectar	1/2 cup orange juice,[a] grapefruit juice[a]
1/2 cup pineapple, canned in its own juice	1 cup peaches, canned in water or own juice
1/2 small banana, grapefruit[a]	1/4 cantaloupe, honeydew
10 cherries	12 grapes
1 cup watermelon, raspberries, strawberries	1/2 cup fruit cocktail, canned in water or natural juice
2 tbsp raisins	2/3 cup blueberries

[a] Vitamin C rich fruits.

If you are dieting, notice that portion sizes are bigger when you eat the whole fruit rather than drink the juice of that fruit. For example, you can have 1/2 cup of grapefruit juice or you can eat 1/2 of a grapefruit. You will feel fuller and more satisfied if you eat the 1/2 of a grapefruit rather than drink a 1/2 cup of juice, even though the calories are the same.

In general, the best buys in this group are those fresh fruits which are in season. See the buying guide for a seasonal chart (pages 172–73) and other tips (beginning on page 166).

Vegetables

Vegetables are the stems, leaves, flowers, roots, or tubers and nonsweet fruits of plants. They are rich in vitamins, minerals, and fiber and low-low in calories (see table 4.4).

Stems are asparagus and celery. Carrots, parsnips, and rutabaga are examples of roots and tubers. Artichokes, broccoli, Brussels sprouts, and cauliflower are flowers. Corn and green beans are seeds. Spinach and lettuce are leaves. And cucumbers, eggplant, and tomatoes are fruits, although they are not sweet.

Government surveys indicate that this is an area of the American diet that needs attention. We eat far too few vegetables and often eat the same ones (corn, green beans, and peas) over and

TABLE 4.4   VEGETABLE GROUP
(Approximately 40 Calories)

½ Cup Raw or Cooked	
Artichoke hearts	Green beans
Asparagus	Kale
Bean sprouts	Onions
Beets	Sauerkraut (rinsed)
Broccoli	Tomato juice (unsalted)
Carrots	Tomatoes
Collard greens	Turnips
Eggplant	Wax beans

1 Cup Raw or Cooked	
Beet greens	Mushrooms
Cabbage	½ cup cooked spinach
Cauliflower	2 cups raw spinach
Cucumbers	Summer squash and zucchini
Green bell peppers	⅓ cup tomato sauce

Unlimited Amounts	
Celery	Radishes
Lettuce	

over. I call this SOS eating . . . the Same Old Stuff. It is no wonder that kids think vegetables are boring; they have only met a few!

In addition to variety, there are important health reasons to expand the number and type of vegetables which your family eats. The National Cancer Institute study on diet and cancer emphasized the benefits of including more vitamin A rich and fiber-filled foods in our diets. Vegetables are the major source of these two nutrients.

Choose at least one dark green leafy vegetable every other day for vitamin A, folic acid, and fiber. And one dark yellow or orange vegetable daily for vitamin A.

As with fruits, the best buys in vegetables are generally those that are in abundant supply. See the buying guide for a seasonal availability chart (pages 172–73) and tips on buying canned and frozen versions (pages 170–75).

Protein Foods

Body-building proteins, some B complex vitamins, and iron are available from these foods. Watch out. These foods can also be high in fat (see table 4.5). Use only the leanest cuts of meat, trim away all visible fat, and remove skin from chicken.

Do not add fat to these foods by frying them. Bake, broil, or poach them. And watch serving size. Remember, other foods also provide small amounts of protein. Americans already eat far more protein than we need (see page 42).

TABLE 4.5 PROTEIN FOODS GROUP
(Approximately 150 Calories)

2 oz cooked *lean* beef (hamburger, steak)
2 oz cooked *lean* pork (1 small chop)
2 oz cooked *lean* chicken without skin (1½ legs, ½ whole breast)
3½ oz tuna (packed in water)
4 oz shrimp
3 oz cod, haddock
5 oz sole, scrod
2 eggs (watch out: 250 mg cholesterol each . . . limit weekly intake)
½ cup cottage cheese (cut calories by using low-fat)
¾ cup cooked dried beans, peas, lentils, or legumes
1½ tbsp peanut butter (less 1 fat allowance)
1½ oz cheese such as Cheddar, American, Gruyère, Swiss, Muenster, Jack, Parmesan[a]

[a] Because cheese is a good source of protein it occurs in both the dairy and protein food groups.

The best meat buys for the buck are the lean cuts. As fat increases so does cost—and calories. Use dried beans, peas, lentils, and other legumes more frequently. Recall from table 2.5, page 43, that they are low in cost, low in fat, and low in calories. The buying guide (page 195) gives other tips to cut costs.

Carbohydrates

This group provides B complex vitamins, iron, and complex carbohydrates. Give preference to unrefined products. They are higher in fiber content, lower in calories, and usually a better buy. (See table 4.6.)

When you do buy refined products, such as pastas, make sure that they are enriched to replace the vitamins and minerals which were lost during processing.

Recall from chapter 2 that these foods are not in and of themselves fattening. But we too often use them as vehicles to carry calorie-loaded toppings to our mouths. A slice of nine-grain bread all warm from the toaster is delicious just as it is and has only about 90 calories. Laden with butter and jam, the calorie count jumps to over 200. Be clear who the culprits are!

TABLE 4.6 CARBOHYDRATE FOOD GROUP
(Approximately 75 Calories)

1 slice bread, whole grain or enriched
1 small dinner roll or biscuit
½ hard roll, hamburger or hot-dog bun, English muffin, bagel
½ medium or 1 small potato, baked or boiled . . . PLAIN
1 small or ½ medium muffin—corn, blueberry, bran
1½ cups popcorn (NO butter or salt!)
1 cube (1½ in. square) corn bread
1 tortilla, 6 in.
1 slice pizza crust (¼ of 10-in. pie)
½ cup cooked cereal, farina, oats, grits, wheat meal
¼ cup granola (high in sugar)
½ cup whole grain brown or white enriched rice, cooked
½ cup cooked whole grain or enriched noodles, macaroni, spaghetti
2 3-in. griddle cakes
5 2-in. square crackers
1 6-in. whole wheat or enriched pita (pocket) bread

The best buys in this group are also the tastiest. Whole grain and less refined products are chewy and filling due to their higher fiber content and often cost less than highly processed choices. See the buying guide (page 181) for pitfalls to avoid in this group.

Fats and Oils

Fats and oils are carriers of fat-soluble vitamins A, D, E, and K, and the essential fatty acids. However, recall from chapter 2 that you need only the equivalent of 2 tablespoons of fat daily to meet these needs. So be very cautious here or the calories can add up quickly (see table 4.7).

Treats

Dollar for dollar, these foods provide little nutrition and lots of calories (table 4.8). They can be a drain on your food budget, robbing your family of important nutrients.

TABLE 4.7 FATS AND OILS GROUP
(Approximately 100 Calories)

1 tsp butter	1 tsp vegetable oil
1 tsp mayonnaise	2 tbsp salad dressing
1 tsp margarine	⅛ of 4-in. avocado
2 tbsp gravy	2 tsp cream cheese
2 tbsp cream sauce	6 small nuts: almonds,
1 tbsp heavy cream	cashews, filberts, etc.
(sweet or sour)	

When you want a treat, reach for a peach, pear, or plum before plummeting your hand into the cookie jar. You will be pennies and pounds wiser. Save these foods for weekends when the family is planning a five-mile bicycle ride so that you can burn the calories before they can take permanent residence in your fat cells.

TABLE 4.8 TREATS GROUP
(Approximately 150 Calories)

Treats	Advice to the Weak of Will!
½ cup ice cream	Notice that frozen yogurt is not
½ cup frozen yogurt	any less fattening than ice cream
¾ cup ice milk	Also note that ice milk has fewer calories and costs less than the other two
5 oz (½ typical serving) milk shake	Better take someone along to drink the other half
1 cup hot chocolate	Only if you skied or raked leaves all day . . . then you could even have a marshmallow on top
1 small serving onion rings	No catsup. Even though a
1 small serving French fried potatoes	president says it is a vegetable, it is 40% sugar
2 small cookies	Not the icing-filled ones
1 brownie	Size 2 in. by 2 in., no icing
1 slice cake	1/16 of 9-in. cake . . . not ¼
1 doughnut	Sugar, plain, or glazed, not the kreme-filled
½ cup pudding or Jell-O	There is not "always room" for extra calories in your diet!
1 oz trail mix	Only if you are traveling the trails with Euell Gibbons

PUTTING IT INTO PATTERNS

Now, let's begin to put menus together. First we need to know how many choices we can have from each food group in order to provide either 1600–1800 calories or 2200–2400 calories. (See table 4.9.) Will we have six dairy food choices and three treats, or three dairy and six treats?

We do not eat all of our protein at one meal and all of our fruit at another. So we next need to decide when we will eat the foods. Will we have fruit at breakfast and as a snack or at lunch and dinner?

TABLE 4.9 DAILY NUMBER OF SERVINGS FROM EACH FOOD GROUP

	No. of Servings	
Food Group	1600–1800 Calories	2200–2400 Calories
Dairy	3	4
Protein	3	4
Fruits	4	5
Vegetables	4	5
Carbohydrates	6	8
Fats and oils	2	4
Treats	Only twice a week for both	

To explain, if you want to eat 1600–1800 calories daily, you will include three dairy food selections in your meals throughout the day. This could be ¾ cup of whole milk in your coffee throughout the day and 3 ounces of cheese as a snack in the midafternoon.

If you plan to eat 2200–2400 calories daily, you will get an additional dairy food selection. So you might have the same ¾ cup of whole milk in your coffee throughout the day, 3 ounces of cheese as a snack, and a cup of yogurt with lunch.

Patterns

The food selections at each calorie level can be eaten in any number of combinations or patterns. As mentioned, surveys show that most people eat in one of three patterns:

Pattern I: 3 meals and 1 snack
Pattern II: 3 meals and 2 snacks
Pattern III: 2 meals and 2 snacks

Following are examples of how to distribute the food selections into these patterns and a sample menu for each. Note that everyone eats the same foods, just in different serving numbers and sizes.

Pattern I: 3 Meals and 1 Snack

This is the traditional pattern of eating and the pattern followed most often by children (tables 4.10 and 4.11). Generally their snack occurs after school, although this could be an evening snack.

As noted in chapter 3, for those who are watching their weight, it is preferable to eat little in the evening and to have a relatively large breakfast or lunch. If dieting, the snack could be eaten midmorning or early afternoon.

TABLE 4.10 PATTERN I: 3 MEALS AND 1 SNACK

Food Groups:	Dairy	Protein	Fruits	Vege-tables	Carbo-hydrates	Fats and Oils
1600–1800 Calories						
Breakfast	1	0	1	0	1	0
Lunch	1	1	2	2	2	0
Dinner	0	2	0	2	2	0
Snack	1	0	1	0	1	1
Total	3	3	4	4	6	2
2200–2400 Calories						
Breakfast	1	0	2	0	2	1
Lunch	2	2	2	2	2	0
Dinner	0	2	0	3	3	2
Snack	1	0	1	0	1	1
Total	4	4	5	5	8	4

Pattern II: 3 Meals and 2 Snacks

This pattern is more common to very small children who have tiny stomachs and must eat small amounts more frequently

TABLE 4.11 SAMPLE MEAL PLAN, PATTERN I

Meal	1800 Serving Size	2400 Serving Size
Breakfast		
Small bran muffin	1	2
Butter	1 tsp	1 tsp
Small orange	1	0
Orange juice	0	8 oz (1 cup)
Skim milk	1½ cups (12 oz)	1½ cups
Lunch		
Sandwich		
Whole wheat pita bread	2	2
Shredded cheese[a]	1½ oz	3 oz
Slices of mushrooms		
Sliced/diced tomato	Enough to make bulging pockets	
Alfalfa sprouts		
Grapes	24	24
Skim milk	1½ cups skim (12 oz)	1½ cups skim
Broccoli flowerets	0	1 cup raw
Dinner		
Sole in wine herb sauce with mushrooms	10 oz	10 oz
Rice pilaf	1 cup	1 cup
Carrots	½ cup	1 cup
Tossed salad	1 cup	1½ cups
Salad dressing	0 (lemon juice)	2 tsp
Hard roll	0	1
Butter	0	1 tsp
Snack		
Strawberries sprinkled with	1 cup	1 cup
granola	¼ cup	¼ cup
light cream	1 tbsp	2 tbsp
Skim milk	1½ cups	1½ cups

[a] Cheese counts as protein not as a dairy on this lunch.

(tables 4.12 and 4.13). Pregnant women may find in the last several months of pregnancy that a pattern of smaller meals like this works well for them.

The snacks can be taken midmorning and midafternoon or midmorning and early evening, or midafternoon and early evening. Again, I recommend eating earlier in the day and avoiding after-dinner snacking.

TABLE 4.12 PATTERN II: 3 MEALS AND 2 SNACKS

Food Groups:	Dairy	Protein	Fruits	Vege-tables	Carbo-hydrates	Fats and Oils
1600–1800 Calories						
Breakfast	0	1	1	0	2	1
Lunch	1	0	1	0	1	0
Dinner	0	2	0	2	2	1
Snack I	1	0	1	2	1	0
Snack II	1	0	1	0	0	0
Total	3	3	4	4	6	2
2200–2400 Calories						
Breakfast	1	1	1	0	2	1
Lunch	1	1	2	1	2	1
Dinner	0	2	0	2	3	2
Snack I	1	0	1	2	1	0
Snack II	1	0	1	0	0	0
Total	4	4	5	5	8	4

Pattern III: 2 Meals and 3 Snacks

This pattern is typical of single adults and teenagers who sleep late and grab their first food rushing to school or work and who tend to stay up later at night (tables 4.14 and 4.15). It is not my favorite pattern, but then again, I was raised in the country where "early to bed, early to rise" was the rule.

VEGETARIANS

Increasingly today, for moral, religious, health, and economic reasons, people are choosing to omit red meat, poultry, and fish from their diets. In many parts of the world, omitting these foods is not a matter of choice but a matter of circumstance. Animal protein is unaffordable and unavailable.

Animal protein is costly. To produce 1 pound of animal protein requires approximately 8–10 pounds of plant protein. Theoretically, animals can be fed plant foods which humans cannot metabolize, thus converting nonusable to usable food for us. While this is possible, it is not common practice in America. Instead, our cattle, poultry, and pork are fed grains, particularly wheat and corn, which could be consumed by humans. This increases the cost of protein production.

TABLE 4.13 SAMPLE MEAL PLAN, PATTERN II

Meal	1800 Serving Size	2400 Serving Size
Breakfast		
Egg, poached	1 medium	1 medium
English muffin	1 whole	1 whole
Butter	1 tsp	1 tsp
Cantaloupe	¼ small	¼ small
Low-fat milk	0	1 cup
Lunch		
Yogurt, plain, mixed with	1 cup	1 cup
blueberries	⅔ cup	⅔ cup
Bran muffin	1 small	0
Sandwich		
Whole wheat bread	0	2 slices
Peanut butter[a]	0	1½ tbsp
Banana (sliced on sandwich)	0	½ small
Dinner		
Chicken cacciatore	4 oz	4 oz
(standard recipe, no fat)		
Noodles	1 cup	1 cup
Zucchini with dill	1 cup	1 cup
Tossed salad	1 cup	1½ cups
Salad dressing	0 (lemon juice)	2 tsp
Italian bread		1 slice
Honeydew melon	¼ small	¼ small
Snack I		
Cheese	1½ oz	1½ oz
Crackers	5 (2 in. sq)	5 (2 in. sq)
Cauliflowerets	1 cup	1 cup
Bell pepper slivers	1 cup	1 cup
Snack II		
Fruit shake[b]		
Low-fat milk	1 cup	1 cup
Frozen blackberries	1 cup	1 cup

[a] Peanut butter counts as 1 protein and 1 fat serving.
[b] Fruit shake: put ingredients in blender and blend until frothy and foamy.

As food costs continue to skyrocket, more and more of us will choose to limit the amount of animal protein in our diets in order to control family food costs. Others are eating less meat to control their intake of fats and cholesterol. The trend toward less animal protein is reflected in U.S. Department of Agricul-

TABLE 4.14 PATTERN III: 2 MEALS AND 3 SNACKS

Food Groups:	Dairy	Protein	Fruits	Vege-tables	Carbo-hydrates	Fats and Oils
1600–1800 Calories						
A.M. snack	1	0	0	0	1	0
Lunch	1	1	0	2	1	1
P.M. snack	1	0	1	0	0	0
Dinner	0	2	1	2	2	1
Night snack	0	0	2	0	1	0
Total	3	3	4	4	5	2
2200–2400 Calories						
A.M. snack	1	0	0	0	2	0
Lunch	1	1	0	2	2	1
P.M. snack	1	0	1	0	0	0
Dinner	1	2	0	3	2	1
Night snack	0	2	2	0	1	0
Total	4	5	3	5	7	2

ture studies which indicate that consumption of red meat, pork, and eggs has declined in the past decade.

People who do not eat meat are called "vegetarians." They can be divided into two types: those who use no animal products at all are called pure vegetarians or vegans, and those who include some milk, dairy products, and eggs in their meals are called lacto-ovo vegetarians. Both patterns have become so popular that today you can order either pure or lacto-ovo vegetarian meals on all commercial airlines.

Lacto-Ovo Pattern

The foods included in the sample Pattern III menu (table 4.15) are typical of a lacto-ovo vegetarian diet. Meal patterns for vegetarians will look no different from meal patterns for those who eat meat. Some vegetarians will have two meals and three snacks daily and others will have three meals and one snack.

The main difference in diet is the food choices included (or excluded), not the pattern in which they are eaten. Vegetarians will omit the meat choices in the protein food group and will instead choose lentils, dried beans and peas, peanut butter, and soybeans.

Because plant proteins have lower levels of one or more of the

TABLE 4.15 SAMPLE MEAL PLAN, PATTERN III

Meal	1800 Serving Size	2400 Serving Size
A.M. snack		
Small blueberry muffin	I	2
Butter	o	I tsp
Whole milk	¾ cup (6 oz)	¾ cup
Lunch		
Spinach and mushroom salad		
Spinach, raw	I cup	I cup
Mushrooms, raw	I cup	I cup
Alfalfa sprouts	½ cup	½ cup
Medium-sized egg, sliced	2	2
Salad dressing	2 tsp	2 tsp
Hard dinner roll	I	2
Whole milk	¾ cup	¾ cup
P.M. snack		
Melted cheese	1½ oz	1½ oz
over torta chips		
made from tortillas, 6 in.	I	2
Grapefruit juice	o	½ cup
Dinner		
Meatless chili beans	1½ cups	1½ cups
Corn bread (1½" square)	2	2
Butter	I tsp	I tsp
Hearty salad tossed with lemon juice		
Broccoli flowerets	½ cup	½ cup
Carrots	¼ cup	½ cup
Radishes	free	free
Cucumbers	½ cup	½ cup
Bell peppers	¼ cup	¼ cup
Whole milk	o	¾ cup
Night snack		
Popcorn	1½ cups	1½ cups
Melted cheese over popcorn	o	3 oz
Orange juice	I cup	I cup

essential amino acids, special attention must be given to the protein in the diet of vegetarians. Lacto-ovo vegetarians will have no problem in assuring that their diets contain a balance of all the essential amino acids. Their diets will include small amounts of milk, dairy products and eggs, each of which provide complete proteins.

Vegans, on the other hand, will need to combine plant proteins to ensure that all the essential amino acids are present simultaneously (table 4.16). This is neither impossible nor difficult, but it requires awareness of combinations. Cereal grain proteins (such as wheat, rice, or corn) are low in lysine (one of the essential amino acids) but contain adequate methionine (another essential amino acid). Therefore, they can be eaten in combination with legumes (such as beans, chick-peas, lentils, and peanuts) which are low in methionine but contain adequate lysine. As explained when we discussed protein, pages 40–46, many of these combinations are traditional and lend themselves to exciting and exotic recipes. For a sampling of good recipes see *Recipes for a Small Planet* by Frances Moore Lappé.

Special attention is also needed for those nutrients which are most abundant in meats and dairy products. Vitamin B-12 is found naturally only in animal products. Vegans may need to use fortified soybean milk or other soy products to ensure adequate B-12 intake. Riboflavin may also be low, so frequent and careful selection of legumes, whole grains, and vegetables is needed.

Getting enough calcium can be a problem for children, and pregnant and lactating women who are pure vegetarians. Calcium is found in dark green leafy vegetables, some nuts (for example, almonds, filberts), legumes, and tofu. These foods must be included daily in the diet.

Iron content may also be marginal. Vitamin C enhances the absorption of iron. Therefore, vegetable sources of iron should be eaten in combination with vitamin C rich foods.

Many of these rules are good advice to us all. Fruit, vegetable, and whole grain sources of important nutrients are considerably lower in fat than are meats and dairy products. Recall that animal foods are our primary source of fats, saturated fats, and cholesterol. Meatless meals make good nutritional sense and can save cents. If you are not vegetarian and do not already do so, you should consider adding at least one meatless day to your family's weekly menus.

Pure Vegetarian Pattern

Notice that the dairy foods group has disappeared and that the protein foods group would contain only the peanut butter, dried beans, peas and legumes, and tofu.

TABLE 4.16 DAILY NUMBER OF SERVINGS

Food Group	1600–1800	2200–2400
Protein	4	5
Fruit	4	5
Vegetables	6	6
Carbohydrates	7	9
Fats/Oils	4	7
Treats	only twice/week for both	

Vegetarian Pattern I: 3 Meals and 1 Snack

Only one vegetarian pattern example will be given (tables 4.17 and 4.18). The others, Patterns II and III, would look just like those for nonvegetarians, except with foods other than animal foods supplying all protein.

TABLE 4.17 VEGETARIAN PATTERN I: 3 MEALS AND 1 SNACK

Food Groups:	Protein	Fruits	Vege-tables	Carbo-hydrates	Fats and Oils
1600–1800 Calories					
Breakfast	1	1	0	2	1
Lunch	1	2	3	2	1
Dinner	2	1	2	2	2
Snack	1	1	1	1	0
Total	5	5	6	7	4
2200–2400 Calories					
Breakfast	1	1	0	2	1
Lunch	2	2	3	2	3
Dinner	2	1	2	3	3
Snack	1	1	1	2	0
Total	6	5	6	9	7

PREGNANCY AND LACTATION

Nutrient needs during pregnancy and lactation increase slightly, not drastically. Pregnancy is neither the time to go whole hog nor to embark on a weight control program.

TABLE 4.18 SAMPLE PURE VEGETARIAN MEAL PLAN

Meal	1600–1800 Serving Sizes	2200–2400 Serving Sizes
Breakfast		
Nine-grain bread	2 slices	2 slices
Peanut butter (subtract 1 fat)	1½ tbsp	1½ tbsp
Fresh peach	1 small	1 small
Lunch		
Vegetarian stir fry		
Carrots	½ cup	½ cup
Broccoli	½ cup	½ cup
Bean sprouts	½ cup	½ cup
Tofu	1 cube	2 cubes
Sesame oil	2 tsp	3 tsp
Rice	1 cup	1 cup
Banana	1 small	1 small
Dinner		
Vegetarian lasagne		
Noodles	1 cup	1 cup
Tomatoes	½ cup	½ cup
Mushrooms	1 cup	1 cup
Red kidney beans	1½ cups	1½ cups
Olive oil	2 tsp	2 tsp
Whole wheat bread	0	1 slice
Soybean margarine	0	1 pat
Poached pears	1 small	1 small
Snack		
Hommos (chick-peas)	¾ cup	¾ cup
Crackers, 2 in. square	5	10
Cucumber spears	1 cup	1 cup
Apple	1 small	1 small

You will be eating for two. However, one of those two is a very small little being that really does not need many calories. Energy requirements increase only by 300 calories during pregnancy. That number is consistent throughout the pregnancy, even during the last months when baby is gaining weight in preparation for birth.

The recommended weight gain for pregnancy is around 24 pounds. It should be gained at a slow and steady pace over the nine months, with more of the gain occurring after the fourth month than before. Studies show that women who gain considerably less weight than this frequently deliver infants of low birth weight.

Pregnancy is absolutely NOT the time to undertake a program to lose weight—no matter what your prepregnancy weight. Drastic restrictions in food intake will reduce the nutritional quality of your diet and risk insufficient supplies of nutrients for your developing baby.

Your commitment should be first and foremost to an adequate and balanced diet. Following such a plan should keep weight gain within normal ranges, even if you began your pregnancy overweight. That is, if you are 5 feet 4 inches and weigh 150 pounds before pregnancy, expect to weigh around 175 pounds at term.

Whether you are slim or chubby when you get pregnant, before you reach full term, you will look fat. It is inevitable! If you just can't stand to look fat, get one of those shirts that say "I'm not fat, I'm pregnant." Then you can at least stop worrying about whether people think you are just fat, and know that they will share your excitement about the coming event.

While babies may start as a twinkle in Daddy's eye, it takes more than that to have them grow and develop normally during pregnancy. They are totally dependent upon you to eat the right foods to meet their nutrient needs. With the possible exception of iron and folic acid, the increased amounts of nutrients needed for pregnancy can be supplied by food. Daily supplements of iron and folate are usually prescribed during pregnancy.

If your diet is well-balanced and adequate before pregnancy, all you will have to do to meet the slightly increased demands of pregnancy is to add a glass of milk, a fresh orange, or other vitamin C rich food, and an additional serving of protein food. These foods will provide the additional calcium, phosphorus, protein, vitamins A and C, and other nutrients required for pregnancy.

Nutrient needs for lactating women are like those for pregnancy plus one more milk or dairy product food added. You will also need to increase your fluid intake to at least 2–3 quarts of liquid daily.

Although we do not write this in professional journals, it is common practice for nutritionists to encourage lactating women to drink a beer while they are nursing. No scientific reason for this. It just seems to help Mom relax and it does add calories and fluid. One is enough!

INFANT FEEDING

I have definite prejudices and will save them for some future exposé rather than to belabor them here. In brief, they are that cow's milk is meant for baby calves and human milk is meant for our babies. Infant formula manufacturers do a marvelous job of copying mother's milk, but it is not "the real thing."

It is a common American myth that many women cannot breast-feed. We are among the healthiest and best nourished people on earth. When we choose to, we can breast-feed. As nutritionist in a clinic for high-risk pregnant women in San Francisco, I worked with 623 women and their infants. All but a small number chose to breast-feed and all who chose to were successful. For reasons of nutrition and health, sanitation, economy, and convenience, I invite and encourage you to breast-feed your next child. Enough said here.

About solid foods for infants: for the first three to four months there is generally no need for foods in addition to breast milk. Baby has a sucking reflex at this stage but no swallowing reflex. If you put food in baby's mouth, baby's tongue thrusts it forward in an attempt to suck it down, and most of the food lands on baby's face and your lap. If you enjoy scooping puree off baby's face, proceed. However, it is unnecessary nutritionally for most infants at this age.

At around 3–4 months, baby's calorie needs can no longer be met by breast milk. Babies need a more concentrated source of calories and also a source of iron and vitamin C. Because God makes no mistakes, it is also at about this time that baby begins to hold ups its head, to sit with minimal support, and to be able to transfer food from the front of the tongue to the back of the mouth and swallow it. No more dribbling down the chin!

Dry cereals, egg yolk in small amounts (it is high in iron but also high in cholesterol), or mashed dried beans, and a bit of juice can now be added. Tofu is a great addition for protein. It is fairly bland in taste, smooth in texture, and easy to digest. By 6–7 months, baby can sit unsupported, balance the head, and begins to smack food in mock chewing motion.

It is about this age that the baby also begins to explore the world orally. Nothing is sacred and everything goes directly into the mouth! Finely chopped, mashed, and strained fruits and vegetables can now be added. Teeth begin to develop and baby will need foods for gumming.

For reasons which I do not know or remember, my grandfather had no teeth . . . and no false teeth. He somehow managed to eat meat, apples, and all sorts of foods which I still believe require teeth. At the age of five I became intensely aware of teeth. My newborn cousin arrived without them and I was quite concerned. How would she ever survive? It was then that I realized that Grandpa had no teeth. I was very upset. What could be done? I worried for weeks about how we could make teeth for her and Grandpa.

It is not necessary to buy special foods for baby. Baby can eat baby cereals or adult cereals like Cream of Wheat, Malt-o-Meal, and eventually, oatmeal. Fruits can be cooked and mashed or fresh ones can be scraped, mashed, or strained.

Table vegetables can be pureed, strained, or mashed. It is easiest to puree a small batch at a time rather than to make each serving individually. Put the excess in ice cubes and freeze. To prepare a meal for baby, simply thaw and heat a cube or two.

If you are using family food, take out an unseasoned portion for baby and do not add sugar, salt, or other seasonings. Babies seem to like the plain, unadorned tastes of foods. In fact, baby food manufacturers for a number of years put salt and sugar in baby foods, but not for baby. Baby didn't care. It was for Mom. Mothers often taste things before offering them to baby. Because she wanted foods to taste well seasoned, manufacturers seasoned them.

Then scientific studies recommended that infants not be given salt or sugar in their foods. Most manufacturers took them out and today most infant foods do not contain salt, sugar, fat, color, or flavor additives or modified starch. Some do still add these ingredients, so read the ingredient information on the label carefully to make sure that they haven't been added.

When the baby boom dried up, the number of babies available to eat baby foods dropped. Manufacturers, who needed to stay in business, looked around to see what they could do with their existing equipment. They invented "toddler" foods. These are, in my opinion, not good buys. There is no reason why a child of this age should not eat table foods.

You are creating work for yourself, not saving work or time, if you are using toddler foods. You must heat them separately and wash the heating container. It is more efficient and economical to mash a bit of the family's food for junior.

PLANNING FAMILY MENUS

Corporations engage in planning activities on a regular basis. They have five-year plans, annual plans, and monthly/weekly plans. Executives of the company meet to agree upon goals, objectives, and strategies. These are broken down into manageable tasks for assignment to staffs, for order of needed supplies, and for setting of time lines. No less is needed in planning family meals.

Set aside a specific time for planning the week's menus. Plan complicated meals for evenings when you will have lots of help or lots of time. Do not plan them for evenings when you expect to be short of time or exhausted from your day's responsibilities.

Plan some meals for preparation by family members who have minimal preparation skills. Your teenagers (both sexes) can prepare fairly complicated meals. Your smaller children can prepare simpler meals.

Select one of the daily meal patterns (I, II, or III) which looks most like the way your family eats. Plan approximate meals for each day based on that pattern. Notice that the patterns include snack meals. These should be planned. They should not occur by accident. Whatever is eaten at these times makes a contribution—which can be negative or positive—to family health and takes a toll on family food budget. Make them count.

When you have planned your menus, check each day for the following:

1. Among the fruits and vegetables planned, is there
   A very good vitamin C source?
      Citrus fruits, strawberries, cantaloupe, cabbage, green peppers, tomatoes, potatoes
   A very good vitamin A source?
      Carrots, sweet potatoes, broccoli, winter squash, apricots, peaches, milk
   A dark green leafy vegetable?
      Spinach, kale, chard, collard, mustard or turnip greens, watercress, parsley
   At least one serving which is raw?
2. Among the carbohydrate foods planned, are they
   Predominantly whole grain products?
   Some enriched or fortified products?

Few highly processed, refined products (crackers, sugary cereals)?
3. Among the dairy foods, are
   Most selected in low-fat or skimmed versions?
   Extra servings included for pregnant and lactating women?
4. Among the protein foods, is there
   At least one meatless meal weekly?
   Only lean, trimmed beef or pork or skinless poultry?
   Fish at least one meal weekly?
   No fried, only broiled, baked, or poached recipes?
5. Is there variety in color, texture, flavor, and aroma?

I've included a planning work section in the Appendix for your use in planning menus.

To get you started, following are seven days of menus, two in each pattern and one vegetarian for your meatless day (tables 4.19 through 4.22). The menus use a wide variety of foods, provide all the essential nutrients your body needs, contain less than 35 percent of the calories in the form of fat, contain no added sugar, and are low-cost.

Serving sizes for each calorie level are not indicated. Refer to the serving sizes listed in each food group beginning on page 263 or in the worksheets in the Appendix beginning on page 259.

SEVEN DAYS OF MENUS

TABLE 4.19 TWO MENUS FOR PATTERN I: 3 MEALS AND
1 SNACK DAILY

Meal	Day One	Day Two
Breakfast	Grapefruit juice Hot oatmeal Butter or margarine Skim milk	Blueberries English muffin Butter or margarine Skim milk

Lunch	Tuna sandwich
	   Whole wheat bread
	   Tuna
	   Lettuce
	   Tomato
	Skim milk
	Honeydew
		Cold pasta salad
		   Shell noodles
		   Cheese chunks
		   Red and green peppers
		   Peas
		Skim milk
		Tangerine

Dinner	Chicken kabobs
	   Chicken chunks
	   Small whole onions
	   Small tomatoes
	Barley
	Spinach salad
	Poppy seed dressing
		Seafood creole
		   Fish chunks
		   Small onions
		   Tomato
		Brown rice
		Cucumber-escarole salad
		Dill dressing

Snack	Pears
	Cheese
		Banana shake
		   Banana and skim milk
		   blended together

TABLE 4.20 TWO MENUS FOR PATTERN II: 3 MEALS AND
2 SNACKS DAILY

Meal	Day One	Day Two
Breakfast	Bran muffin Peanut butter Banana (on peanut butter) Low-fat milk	French bread Soft cheese Baked apple Low-fat milk
Lunch	Cottage cheese[a] Pineapple Crackers	Egg sandwich Bread Egg salad made with parsley, mayonnaise and celery Cantaloupe Skim milk
Dinner	Lamb stew Lamb Carrots Celery Onions Potatoes Tossed salad Radishes, oil and vinegar Hard rolls	Bean loaf Pinto beans Bread crumbs Nuts Cheese Tomato paste Tossed salad Tomato and red pepper Green beans
Snack I	Cheese Raw vegetables Bread sticks	Yogurt dip Raw vegetables Toast corners
Snack II	Skim milk Tart apple	Skim milk Fresh peach

[a] By combining the milk and protein servings allowed here, you can have a larger serving of cottage cheese and an easy meal to carry along on the go.

TABLE 4.21 TWO MENUS FOR PATTERN III: 2 MEALS AND 3 SNACKS DAILY

Meal	Day One	Day Two
A.M. snack	Bagel Cream cheese Skim or low-fat milk	Cracked wheat bread Butter or margarine Skim or low-fat milk
Lunch	Chinese stir-fry Snow peas Water chestnuts Bamboo shoots Tofu Long-grain rice Low-fat milk	Chicken-vegetable soup 3–5 vegetables Low-fat broth 2–3 oz chicken chunks Bran muffin Low-fat milk
P.M. snack	Graham crackers Skim or low-fat milk Grapes	Pretzel Cheese Apricot
Dinner	Cuban casserole Black beans Rice and cheese Tossed salad Asparagus	Chicken Marengo Chicken Tomatoes Olives Egg noodles Tossed salad Green beans
Night snack	Corn muffin Juicy peach	Italian bread Hard cheese Unsweetened grape juice

Note: Day One in the pattern above is a lacto-ovo pattern which includes dairy products but not meats.

**TABLE 4.22 ONE DAY OF PURE VEGETARIAN IN PATTERN I:
3 MEALS AND 1 SNACK**

Meal	Day One
Breakfast	Fresh sliced fruit Banana nut bread Sesame butter
Lunch	Tofu burger Burger bun Raw vegetables Pear nectar
Dinner	Soybean stew Soybeans, tomato, onion, celery bell peppers and seasoning Brown rice Baked acorn squash Mixed melon balls
Snack	Fruit shake Tofu, raspberries blended Whole wheat crackers

5. Contingency Plans

Life is full of chance events, changes in circumstances, and both planned and unplanned occurrences. Eating is like that too. There may be days when you grab two snacks instead of your usual lunch; when unexpected guests arrive for dinner and there is nothing to cook; when you are eating out and faced with calorie-tempting choices; and when the recipe you are dying to prepare is clad in a cloak of salt, fat, and sugar.

Corporations have staffs with the responsibility to anticipate, foresee, and predict out-of-the-ordinary occurrences. Much of their work revolves around the question "What if . . ."

In the normal course of business, production occurs on schedule and without variation. To avoid disruption of production and potential financial loss, corporations must anticipate and plan for unusual occurrences. These are called contingency plans.

You will need contingency plans too. They will provide guidelines for what to do when a "What if . . ." event occurs.

SNACKING

According to Mr. Webster, a snack is a "hurried or light meal." However, we act as if the definition of snack was the continuous act of searching for food. We forage for food throughout the day, paying little attention to what we find, as long as we can continue to stuff it into our mouths. Snacks can be light meals, hurriedly eaten, and excellent sources of nutrients. It all depends on the choices we make. It would be foolish to pretend that snacking was not going to occur and to omit it in your planning.

Snacks should be scheduled just like any other meal. Children and adults should be trained to eat at regular periods rather than eating on impulse or continuously. Impulse eaters rarely respond to hunger pangs. Instead they respond to food stimulus. They cannot pass a newsstand without buying a candy bar or an ice-cream store without stopping for a scoop. They are rarely actually hungry because their mouths are rarely empty.

The practice of snacking while on the run has another major drawback. One rarely pays attention to what is being eaten if it is eaten while walking down the street, watching television, riding in a car, or studying for exams. It is not surprising that part of the satisfaction of eating is missed when concentration is distracted. The result is that in a short time the distracted snacker goes foraging for yet another goody.

Serve snacks as if they were meals. Serve them away from other activity locations. Do not combine other activities with eating. Pay attention to the food being eaten. Most snacks take less than five minutes to consume so there is no great time lost to step away from distractions and enjoy the break being taken.

While at work, walk away from your desk for a snack, even if you have carried snack foods to work with you. If you have an employee dining room, lounge, or outdoor sitting area, take your snack there. The break from your work will restore your concentration and freshness when you return to your desk. It will also assure that your attention is on enjoying the foods which you are eating.

If your children like to have a snack when they arrive home from school, which most little people do after a day of study and play, plan for it. Have foods available which are simple to prepare and serve so that they can get their own snack.

Children can make Popsicles from fruit juice. They can make fruit or vegetable shish kabobs from chunks of fruit or vegetable. Each can be dipped in a yogurt sauce. Often children who will not eat cooked vegetables at a meal will eat raw vegetables as a snack.

Finger foods like unsalted nuts and seeds, fresh and dried fruits, whole wheat bread with cheese or peanut butter, fruit juices, and milk are all easy for a child to organize. They are also easy to pack in lunch bags for you or family members to carry to work or school.

If you or a family member has a weight problem, you may want to assemble the snack on a small plate or tray, controlling the portion sizes. It is easier for any of us to stop eating when the plate is clean than to stop when there are still nuts or cookies in the jar.

Our environment today abounds with snack foods. Vending machines, corner newsstands, and checkout counters offer brightly packaged goodies which cry out for your attention. To avoid responding to their pleas, you may want to keep emergency foods at your workplace to eat if you really do get hungry. I like to keep a basket of fresh fruit on my desk which I replenish weekly. You can put unsalted nuts, dried fruits like raisins and apricots, or a jar of peanut butter and some crackers in your desk drawer.

Do not be an accomplice to other people's nutritional crimes. If it is common for doughnuts, coffee cake, pastries, homemade cakes, and other sweet-tooth treats to be left for the forager in the employee lounge or kitchen, pass them by. An occasional piece of cake to celebrate a fellow worker's birthday is one thing. Daily indulgences in sugarly delights are yet another.

If you feel that you cannot resist "just one," then take your break elsewhere or carry in your own snack food. A small piece of fresh fruit has approximately 40 calories. A plain, cake-type doughnut has 100, and a glazed one has over 200. That "harmless" sliver of chocolate cake with icing can have close to 150 calories. It is just not worth it to indulge.

Think of snacking as an important chance to add more nutrients rather than as a deed for which you will later feel regret. Look forward to your snack and be sure that the foods available for snacks and the amount eaten fit within the serving sizes for the menu pattern which is being followed. For example, if following Pattern II, the food choices for a midday snack include one serving of dairy, fruit, and carbohydrate and two vegetable choices. This could be cottage cheese with pineapple and carrot sticks and crackers. Or it could be a mushroom and cheese sandwich with a fresh orange.

Snack foods should be as healthy as mealtime foods. Watch out for foods which add calories but few nutrients to your intake. It is easy to spot them. They are:

○ Greasy-crisp or oily, like snack chips, fried foods
○ Smooth and thick, like peanut butter, cream cheese, cream and sour creams, sauces and gravies, milk shakes, pudding
○ Sweet and gooey, like ice cream, candy, cakes with icing, bakery-type packaged snack cakes and cookies, especially cream-filled ones

Do not confuse snacks with treats. Snacks should be regular, wholesome foods, not cakes and cookies. Dollar for dollar, regular foods provide more nutrition than treat foods do. See the comparison of chips and cookies to vegetables and fruits on page 169.

BAGGING IT

My husband, Steven, forgets to eat lunch if I don't send one with him. Or, if he does remember, he buys what he considers to be a balanced meal—a slice of pizza for one hand and a beer for the other! Rather than beg him not to eat the same thing day after day (I have my reputation to protect!), I pack his lunch.

I also pack a lunch for me when I am working away from my office at home. When I am on the road for a television shoot or scheduled heavily with appointments with clients with whom I do consulting work, I, too, often forget to eat.

Bagged lunches seem far more convenient and time efficient than purchased meals. I can eat when I have a moment rather than requiring time to go to a place to purchase lunch. The remainder of my lunch break can be used for a brisk walk, to window-shop, or to catch up on errands.

Packed lunches are also a great money saver. A deli sandwich can range from $1.50 to over $3.00. Beverages, salad, and fruit add further to the cost. A packed lunch can include a sandwich or leftovers, and rarely costs more than $1.50 for the entire contents of the bag.

Finally, unless you choose very cautiously, lunches eaten out can add excess calories. It is possible to select wisely and keep your waistline trim. We will see how to do that. But first we will look at what to pack in lunches for office and school.

Sandwiches

Sandwiches are the mainstay of our bagged lunches. My cousin calls them "meals with edible napkins," since the bread holds the filling. The trick to great sandwiches is variety. A white bread with bologna and American processed cheese every day deadens the senses. (It also adds excess salt and fat, unnecessary nitrates, and a low-fiber carbohydrate!)

Variety is the key. Even the same basic ingredients can be mixed and matched to form an endless array of sandwich surprises. For example, I use tuna (water-packed) weekly but vary the ingredients mixed with it. One week it may contain the traditional mayonnaise, celery, onion, and chopped egg. The next it will be mixed with oregano and chopped parsley. Then with curry and walnuts (stuffed into pita bread). Or chopped black olives and onion.

We all love peanut butter. It can show up on celery or between crackers. It appears with sliced bananas or raisins or jam. If I make peanut butter and honey sandwiches, I mix the two together then spread it on the bread. That way the honey does not drip out, leaving a trail for bears to follow!

I use a variety of cheeses from plain to fancy. Because cheese is high in fat, I slice it thin and add lots of greens to the sandwich. Mustard makes a tangy condiment with cheese. Grated cheese can be mixed with chutney, curry and nuts, olives, or low-fat cottage cheese. It can also be mixed with drained, mashed beans or tofu for a low-fat/low-calorie filling.

Many leftover main dishes can be turned into sandwich filling. Chicken or turkey can be made into salad either to stuff a pita, a tomato, or a bell pepper or to fill a sandwich. Meat loaf can be chilled, then sliced for a filling. Fish fillets can be garnished with a lemon-yogurt sauce for a fishwich.

Variety in breads also adds interest. I buy several types of bread and store them in the freezer. Each day gets a different selection. We like nine-grain and whole grain breads for cheese, peanut butter, and tofu sandwiches. I also keep pumpernickel and rye, raisin, and Italian breads. Pita, the Middle Eastern pocket bread, is a favorite. It can be stuffed with any sandwich filling and has room for lots of vegetables too. We like a vegetarian pita with sliced mushrooms, shredded carrots, broccoli flowerets, and a yogurt dressing.

When I make cornmeal or bran muffins, I make a double batch. The leftovers are frozen to use in lunches. They make a great addition to lunches which are to be heated, such as soups and stews. They are also a good filler for between-meal snacks.

Sandwiches do not leave my kitchen without lots of greens. Steven claims that he sometimes has to sit on his sandwich first to get it flat enough to fit in his mouth! I keep three types of lettuce on hand and stuff handfuls into each sandwich. We have alfalfa sprouts when I remember to grow them. And periodically, just for fun, I even put in Chinese bean sprouts.

If I am in a particularly "creative" mood, we get "kitchen sink" sandwiches, made of whatever is left over: cooked carrots or other vegetables, sliced and pressed onto cheese; bean and noodle casserole sliced.

Most sandwiches can be made in advance and frozen. Leftover turkey, roast beef, meat loaf, or vegetarian loaf freeze well. Wrap the sandwiches tightly before freezing so that they do not dry out. Do not put mayonnaise on the bread; it tends to separate when frozen. And do not add lettuce or tomatoes. They will change texture when thawed. Instead, send them along in a separate wrap or sandwich bag. Frozen sandwiches will thaw in 3–4 hours at room temperature.

Leftovers

Leftovers do not always hide between bread slices. Steven's office has a a kitchenette, so on occasion I send leftover meals from the night before, assembled like a TV dinner, for him to heat in the toaster oven. Leftovers are economical and a change of pace from sandwiches.

Small glass jars, about 1 cup, can carry pasta salad, yogurt with nuts and fruit, fruit salad, and items to be reheated. Soups, stews, Mexican beans, and casseroles are especially welcome on cold days.

Plastic containers with tight-fitting lids work best for children. Used yogurt, cottage cheese, or margarine tubs work and can be thrown out after this use.

Beverages

I carry a thermos bottle for coffee (my one bad addiction). The thermos is stainless steel—in and out. It is the kind that construction workers use so that they can drop it six stories and still use it the next day. I am a bit clumsy.

Coffee from a vending machine is undrinkable and costs 25 cents per cup minimum. Coffee from the corner coffee shop costs at least 50 cents per cup and varies in quality. I grind my own coffee, use expensive French roast beans, and make an entire thermos of coffee (4 cups) for 27 cents.

Jennifer's lunchbox has its own thermos. I wash it at night with dinner dishes and stick it in the refrigerator. This helps prechill it to keep her juice extra cold the next day.

Other Tricks

If I don't put "zippers" on oranges, they don't get eaten. "Zippers" are made by scoring the orange with a knife in quarters, just deep enough to cut through the skin and pulp. The orange peel comes off easily in four pieces.

A variety of fruits is added to lunch . . . never the same apple a day. At least four different fruits are purchased each week then rotated between lunch and snacks. In the summer, even berries are put in, usually in a container since they crush easily.

I add funny cartoons and articles to the bag. And some days, I hide "love notes" to let my lunchers know that they are loved and cared for.

Costs

If you pack lunches, be aware that costs can skyrocket if you purchase individual servings of foods. Compare:

6 oz can of orange juice	36.5 cents
6 oz of orange juice in thermos	20.4
1 oz individually wrapped cheese slice	13.3
1 oz cheese, sliced by hand	10.8
1 oz box of raisins	16.5
1 oz raisins in plastic bag	1.9

Lunch meats are also expensive. Smoked chicken breast at 74 cents for a 3-ounce package costs $3.92 per pound. Whole chicken breasts sell for not more than $1.19 per pound. In addition to the cost, most lunch meats contain added salt, preservatives, and color and flavoring agents. If you use meat in sandwiches, purchase slightly more fresh meat than you need for meals to guarantee leftovers for lunch boxes.

School Lunches

When my stepdaughter is with us, I make the same sandwiches we eat, but under stricter rules—hers not mine. For example, she likes her peanut butter and jelly sandwiches made inside out. That is, jelly on the bread first, then the peanut butter. She likes mustard instead of mayonnaise, but only on one side.

Children have many unexplainable habits. They will eat the center of the sandwich and bring the dried-out crust home in their lunch box. They will trade your oatmeal-raisin-bran-and-sunflower-seed cookies for cream-filled, sticky, chocolate-coated ones. They will eat their lunch on the way to school, forget it on the bus, or toss it out the window during a head-hitting game. Or they carry it home, uneaten, squashed, and without any recollection of why they forgot to eat lunch.

You may want to consider the school lunch program for your child. Check the weekly menus. Most schools either send menus home with the children or print them in local newspapers. The menus are planned to meet one-fourth of the child's RDA. So you need not worry about how well balanced they are nutritionally. However, depending on how they are prepared and presented, the meals may or may not be appetizing. If your child does not eat the meal because it looks and tastes bad, it does him or her no good.

We loved school lunch as children. Mrs. Covello prepared delicious and wholesome meals for almost three generations of children at Delhi Elementary School. Her chili beans were the best. She always made enough for seconds and we licked the pots clean.

The price of a school lunch will vary by school district depending on local food and labor costs and the amount of reimbursement provided by the district to subsidize the program. In many cases, the cost will be less than the cost of preparing a bag lunch.

A school lunch is certainly a better buy than a bag lunch containing a bologna sandwich on white, spongy bread, a bag of chips, a can of pudding, and a can of punch. The nutrient content of such a bag lunch is marginal, with a glut of negatives like color and flavor additives, preservatives, salt, and sugar.

Dieter's Brown Bag

There is no great mystery to packing a dieter's lunch or keeping on your diet while eating lunch out. Stick to the meal plan provided in the meal pattern guide which you have selected, and keep a keen eye out for hidden calories.

If you are bagging it, select foods within each group which can be packed. Sandwiches are a great dieter's lunch. Bread is not fattening if it is not dripping with mayonnaise or stacked high with fatty pastrami or other high-calorie filling. Two slices of bread will provide you with essential B-vitamins and bulk for a little over 150 calories.

It is what and how much you put between the bread which adds calories. One serving from the protein foods group is 1½ ounces (NOT 2 or 3 or 4 ounces) of cheese. Most cheeses are high in fat. Or it is 2 ounces of *lean* chicken or meat. It is not a pile of fatty corned beef and it is not chicken salad made with 1 ounce of chicken and ¼ cup of mayonnaise.

Dressings, mayonnaise, butter or margarine, and sandwich spreads are full of fat. No need to put these on your sandwich. If you would like a dash of flavor, add mustard. For moisture, add a slice of tomato.

Make your sandwiches irresistible in appearance. Pile them high with bright, crisp lettuce, spinach, or watercress. Stuff alfalfa sprouts or sliced mushrooms in them. These are all low in calories and will add texture, color, flavor, and moisture.

If you tire of sandwiches, carry low-fat yogurt or low-fat cottage cheese mixed with pieces of fresh fruit. Or a light vegetable soup to warm you on a cold day. Or a portion of last night's leftovers. Or a mixed greens and raw vegetable salad with a lemon to squeeze over it for dressing.

The foods which a dieter can carry in a bag lunch are little different from the foods which a dieter would eat if preparing a meal at home. Include lots of crisp and crunchy raw vegetables to fill you up, satisfy your desire to chew and gnaw, and keep your fingers and mouth busy longer. And fresh fruit for a sweet finish.

DIETING OUT

Each year Americans increase the number of meals eaten away from home. We no longer take all of our meals together. Our husbands eat lunch out rather than come home or carry one. Our children may grab meals on the way to and from athletic practices, music lessons, and club meetings. We, too, are no longer home-bound and increasingly eat meals out.

For the single woman, meals eaten away from home may represent the day's major food intake. A business lunch or a dinner date may be the most important meal of the day.

Whether we cook the food or someone else does, the same basic nutritional guidelines apply. We need to select a wide variety of foods to ensure that we get all the essential nutrients needed and balance our intake of macronutrients (fats, carbohydrates, protein) to avoid negative health risks associated with excesses.

When eating out your willpower will face extra tests of strength. A menu full of delicious-sounding entrées has added allure when you do not have to prepare it or clean up afterward. Yet it is possible to eat out regularly without gaining weight. Be alert to potential pitfalls and easy deceptions. A so-called "dieter's plate" (table 5.1) offered by many restaurants can have as many calories as a hamburger.

TABLE 5.1 CALORIES IN DIETER'S PLATE

Dieter's Plate	Calories
3-oz hamburger patty	235
peach half, heavy syrup	100
½ cup regular cottage cheese	110
four saltine crackers	50
Total	495

By comparison, a McDonald's quarter pounder has 424 calories; a Burger King cheeseburger has 350 calories; Arby's Ham 'n' Cheese is 380 calories; a Moby Jack at Jack in the Box is 455 calories; and a Kentucky Fried crispy breast has 286 calories.

An occasional Big Mac will not destroy your diet. That is, if you do not have an order of fries and a shake along with it. However, most fast foods are high in fat and salt, low in fiber, and, with the exception of protein, low in major essential nutrients. Better to visit an establishment with a wider selection of foods than to go "where the beef is" on a regular basis.

A salad bar offers a great option for lunchtime waist watchers. But be careful what you pile on your plate or you will be sabotaged rather than slenderized (table 5.2).

TABLE 5.2 CALORIE COMPARISON OF SALADS

Sabotage Salad	Calories	Slenderizing Salad	Calories
Lettuce, 2 cups of mixed greens	20	Lettuce, 2 cups of mixed greens	20
Marinated beans, ½ cup	110	Raw broccoli, ½ cup	10
Potato salad, ½ cup	165	Shredded carrots, ½ cup	25
Croutons, ½ cup	110	Beets, ½ cup	45
Dressing, 2 tbsp	165	Lemon juice, 2 tsp	10
Total	570	Total	110

A good rule of thumb is to stick to the things which are fresh and plain. Shredded cabbage is all but calorie free. Coleslaw bathing in a mayonnaise dressing is not. A ½ cup plain boiled potato cubes has around 50 calories. A ½ cup of potato salad has 125 calories.

One tablespoon of dressing contains, on the average, 75–80 calories. A fourth of a cup, the amount usually poured on top, contains approximately 300–325 calories. Always put the dressing on the side. When ordering a salad, ask the waiter or waitress to serve it separately. This will allow you to use very small amounts and to distribute it throughout the salad rather than to have it smother the top and disappear before you reach the bottom.

Better yet, ask for oil and vinegar or fresh lemon. Use very little oil: it contains about 100–120 calories per tablespoon. You will soon discover that you love these lighter salads. You can actually taste the individual flavors of the crisp vegetables.

When ordering a plate meal, ask the waiter or waitress what is included with the meal. If you have a choice of type of potato, choose the plain and simple one. French fries and mashed potatoes both have more calories than plain boiled or baked potatoes. Be sure to tell the waiter or waitress to leave off the sour cream, butter, sauce, and gravy.

It is also often possible to make substitutions. Ask if you can have a plain salad instead of the cream soup. If mashed potatoes are the only form of potato offered that day, ask if you can substitute plain rice.

Many foods are cooked plain and then have sauce, gravy, or melted butter poured over them just before serving. For example, vegetables are cooked plain to preserve their color and texture. They are held at serving temperature until ordered. Fish and poultry are often cooked plain. The cook adds butter, sauce, or gravy just before serving. Ask the waiter or waitress to tell the cook to leave them off.

Stick to food choices and portion sizes which match the number of servings and types of foods allowed on the menu pattern which you are following. If portion sizes offered are too large, ask a friend to join you for lunch to split a meal with you. You will both eat half as much for half the price.

Finally, do not play innocent victim. Do not order a meal and then sigh with resignation and eat the whole thing, globs of salad dressing, a sour-cream-covered potato, fried chicken, dessert, and all. Just because someone else is cooking the meal does not mean that you are helplessly condemned to eating an extra 500 calories. Ask what the meal includes, how it is prepared, and what options you have or substitutions you can make to reduce the calories.

These same rules apply to eating dinner out. Select simply prepared menu items and omit the extras. Many restaurants are offering nouvelle or spa cuisine designed especially to appeal to the palate without tripping the scales.

If you like a drink before dinner or wine with your meal and you are watching calories, go lightly. Drinks made with fruit juice base and sugar syrups, such as planter's punch or mai tai, and those made with cream, such as an Alexander or eggnog, can add calories quick. Instead choose a wine spritzer (wine and seltzer), Bloody Mary (tomato juice and vodka or gin), or a nonalcoholic drink like mineral or seltzer water with a twist of lime.

If two of you are dining alone, consider ordering only one glass of wine apiece or a half rather than a full bottle of wine. A dieter's dinner and determination can be destroyed by 110 calories per glass of wine. In addition to the extra calories, alcohol can loosen your resolve to restrain eating.

"IT CANNOT WORK FOR ME BECAUSE MY LIFE DOES NOT LOOK LIKE THAT!"

You may have been reading along thus far and thinking, That is all well and good for her, but my life does not look that way. None of this will work for me. I have more out-of-the-ordinary occurrences than I have routine.

If your eating pattern looks like a series of last-minute responses to crises it is precisely because you have no plan. You are forever trapped in catch-up remedies—the crash diet to undo months of overeating, the vitamin supplement to overcome missed meals and repetitive menus, the ten-day self-improvement plan which gets unbearably boring by the third day.

Several years of crisis eating and you begin to think that your bad habits are normal. It is difficult to see that you have other options. It is difficult to believe that planning, including planning for emergencies, can result in positive health benefits.

The transformation from victim of circumstance to master of nutrition and health is not impossible or even a struggle. Patients I see privately regularly cross the line—with little effort. I will relate a few stories as examples, using pseudonyms.

Marilyn

Marilyn, 31, married, no children, is a clothing designer in New York City. She comes from a Midwestern family with a tendency toward overweight. Although she runs regularly, she weighed 15 pounds more than the standard for her height.

Several habits were contributing to this. She ate no proper breakfast or lunch but grabbed quick hunger-pang killers—a bran muffin and coffee, a slice of pizza. By late afternoon she was famished and would stave off the pains with cookies, an ice-cream cone, peanuts, or a package of crackers and cheese.

At 8:00 P.M. she would meet her husband at a local restaurant, exhausted and starved. (They ate no meals at home . . . not atypical for young New Yorkers.) After a glass of wine, they would order dinner. Nothing exceptional, but in large portions and always with a dessert. If they did not order dessert, her husband, a naturally thin man, would pick up a pint of ice cream on the way home and they would share it before going to bed within the hour.

Marilyn's major problem was that she took in no nutrients or calories during the day when she needed them. She ate most of her food at night, then slept on it. And ate foods which were high in fat content—including her before-bed snack of ice cream.

Her pattern of eating was essentially three meals and two snacks—eaten in the morning, around noon, late afternoon, dinnertime, and before bed. We worked with this pattern—a basic Pattern II menu plan.

At first Marilyn was terrified. It looked to her as if she would be eating much more food than she was accustomed to. We added a fresh fruit and low-fat milk to her morning bran muffin. We structured a lunch pattern which included one choice each of protein and carbohydrate and two vegetables. Her afternoon snack switched from concentrated sweets to a dairy, fruit, and carbohydrate food. Instead of a scoop of ice cream, she now enjoyed yogurt or milk, a piece of fresh fruit, and a few crackers. These could all be easily and quickly purchased and eaten.

Marilyn was no longer tired, listless, and irritable in the late afternoon. At dinner she was no longer famished and could comfortably order foods which followed her meal plan. Before bed she mixed up a "smoothie" (one fruit choice, frozen! and one dairy choice) to join her husband in his "dessert time."

Carolyn

Carolyn, 26, mother of two, married, is a keypunch operator for a utilities company. Following each pregnancy she retained 10 pounds. She was 20 pounds overweight when she came to see me. Her baby is 3½ years old. Her older child is 6 and in first grade.

When introducing herself to me, she emphatically stated that she absolutely never eats and could not understand why she could not lose weight. Carolyn was a classical example of someone without plans whose life is a response to contingencies.

Carolyn's mornings were chaos. She would pack a lunch for her husband, dress the 3½-year-old, and supervise her 6-year-old. By 8:15 A.M. the two children and husband would have had breakfast, prepared by her husband. Carolyn used "breakfast" time to get herself dressed. All would then leave together to be dropped off at school, baby-sitter, commuter train.

Carolyn grabbed coffee (with two sugars) and a newspaper on

the way to the train. Thirty minutes later she arrived at her office where doughnuts are "kindly provided by the management." Carolyn ate two with her second cup of coffee (with two sugars).

Midmorning she felt blah and went to the soda machine for a can of soda. Her lunch break is scheduled for 12:30. Her company has a cafeteria but she hates standing in lines. Besides, she was "dieting" so she did not want to eat a meal. Instead, she grabbed a small package of cookies and a soda, just to tide her over.

Needless to say, by 3:30 P.M. she was starving. Again, with iron will, Carolyn avoided eating a real meal, which she considered to be fattening, and instead had just a "small" candy bar to perk her up and a soda to wash it down.

At five o'clock, she dashed for the train. Passing a newsstand on the way, she would often stop for a bag of chocolate-coated peanuts or a peanut butter cup to get her through until dinner.

At home, she nibbled and sampled as she prepared dinner. A tablespoon or two of Jell-O salad, a lick of the butter knife, several mouthfuls of spaghetti sauce, a sliver of bread as she sliced it for the basket. At the table she served herself small portions or none at all, complaining that she was not hungry. Then as she cleared the table, Carolyn devoured every last morsel of uneaten food.

Carolyn's biggest hurdle was to recognize that she was eating! She just was not eating meals. Her average daily caloric intake was over 2800. Her requirements were in the range of 1800 to 2000. As with Marilyn, the first obstacle with Carolyn was to get her to follow a meal pattern and EAT meals.

Carolyn loved food and was amazed and delighted to begin to EAT. Her dependency on sugar (in coffee, doughnuts, soft drinks, and candy) disappeared "miraculously" when she began to eat simple, wholesome meals. She followed Pattern I: 3 meals and 1 snack.

She got up 10 minutes earlier to allow time to fix her husband's lunch (and one for herself), supervise and dress the children, dress herself, and sit down for 10 minutes to enjoy the breakfast her husband prepared.

Fortified with a good breakfast, she no longer craved double doses of sugar in her coffee and a sweet doughnut fix at the office. Neither did she need a sugared soft drink for a pick-me-up in the late morning.

By carrying a lunch from home, she avoided the cafeteria lines —except on those days when she wanted a soup or fresh salad to supplement it. She also ate foods which contributed essential nutrients and not just empty calories.

While her lunch was substantial, she still wanted a snack for the ride home. An extra piece of fruit carried in her lunch provided the munch and crunch to which she had grown accustomed at 5:00 P.M.

Carolyn now ate dinner with the family. She stopped snitching from the pot before dinner and licking the plates afterward.

Not surprisingly, these changes were easy to institute. Within a week of "eating," Carolyn began to feel less resentful and guilty about food. Her energy level perked up and her craving for sugar-filled foods tapered off. Within four months she had reached her weight goal and has had no further difficulty keeping weight off.

The point is that healthful eating does not require drastic and impossible changes in your life-style. Marilyn and Carolyn did not change the way they lived. They did not suddenly reject their old friends and family, start eating sprouts and nuts, wear funny-looking clothes, and mumble strange-sounding syllables. Neither has any of my other patients.

They have all simply incorporated good, wholesome, and nutritious foods into their existing day-to-day patterns of living. They have substituted good habits for less healthy ones.

They are no longer willows in the wind, bending to the slightest disruption or turbulence. They each have selected a meal pattern which reflects their life-style and supports their nutritional and health goals. They each are able to manage out-of-the-ordinary events without losing control and returning to old habits. They each rave about how good they feel and how easy it is to eat healthfully when you do feel so good as a result. And they each exclaim how they Cannot Believe that They are Eating SO Much! without gaining weight.

THE FINAL FRONTIER

You have finally got it down to a science and an art. You have selected a meal pattern which fits your life-style. You remember the food selections and portion sizes for each meal. It has all become easy and automatic. You are on the road to excellence.

Just as you begin to feel secure, even perhaps a bit smug, your

mother-in-law shows up on a Saturday afternoon and decides to stay for dinner, and there is nothing in the house to cook. Or your favorite niece returns from medical school to announce that she will become a cardiologist and asks if and how you control fat, sugar, and salt in your recipes.

Mother Hubbard's Cupboard

The best-laid plans of mice and men are not without challenges, and even the most organized kitchen manager will on occasion find herself short of time to shop, faced with unexpected guests, or not in the mood to prepare the meal planned.

For those with a bit of imagination, Mother Hubbard's bare cupboard may offer as many surprises as a goose laying golden eggs. Here are some examples of main dishes we have had when there seemed to be nothing to cook. My husband calls these "Depression Della's Dinners."

Note that some of the ingredients used are staples which I always have on hand. They are in the cupboard not as a part of the planned week's menus, but as backups for emergencies. Many of the other ingredients are just what was on hand or left over or unused.

Necessity is truly the mother of invention. You will be amazed at the fabulous meals you can create from nothing when there are unexpected dinner guests. Add a tossed salad and some fresh fruit to these combinations and the meal will be complete.

Mexican Meal: Huevos Rancheros for Four

Tortillas from the freezer; 1 can refried beans; 4 eggs; a bit of shredded cheese; tomato salsa. Heat tortillas. Heat beans. Fry eggs. Assemble each serving as follows: On top of tortilla, place ¼ of the beans, shredded cheese, top with fried egg. Offer salsa for those who like hot sauce.

Italian Meal 1: Pasta Primavera for Four

Cook any type or combination of types of pasta for four. In a separate saucepan, prepare a basic cheese sauce—any recipe, using any suitable cheese. Add several precooked vegetables to sauce . . . any one will do—peas, green beans, carrots, tomato, whatever your vegetable bin contains or was left over from another meal.

Drain pasta, toss with primavera sauce and vegetables.

Italian Meal 2: Pasta del Mar for Four—White and Red

White

Cook any spaghetti, linguini, vermicelli, or mix of them for four. In separate pan, sauté 3–4 minced garlic cloves until tender. Add 1 can of drained clams and toss with drained pasta.

Serve with a vegetable in addition to the salad.

Red

This can also be made as a red clam sauce. Toss clams and pasta with from 1 to 1½ cups marinara sauce (we make it in huge batches, separate into jars, seal, and store for up to one month in the refrigerator).

Terrific Tuna

Tuna can become a luncheon salad niçoise with fresh green beans and boiled potato arranged on a bed of lettuce with a light vinaigrette dressing.

It can be the standard tuna and noodle casserole recipe found in any cookbook.

It can be mixed with eggs and cheese, poured into a pastry shell, and voilà, tuna quiche.

Or mix tuna with peas and egg, form into four balls. Place each ball in the middle of a square of crescent roll dough (do not divide the dough on the diagonal). Roll, place on a cookie sheet, and bake until the rolls are done. Serve with a sauce of yogurt seasoned with a little lemon and parsley.

Oriental Stir Fry

You do not need bean sprouts and snow peas to make an Oriental Stir Fry. Like thrifty homemakers in the Orient, you can use whatever is available.

Prepare rice for four–½ cup per person before cooking is usually enough.

In a skillet or wok, add oil (preferably sesame or peanut but any oil will do). Toss in chopped onion or garlic, fresh ginger or a tasty amount of powdered ginger. Sauté whatever vegetables are available: celery, broccoli, carrots, peppers, spinach, or other dark greens, squash . . . whatever. After approximately 5 minutes, add a mixture of 1 tablespoon cornstarch, ¼ cup soy sauce, 1 teaspoon sugar. Toss with vegetables until the sauce thickens and serve over the rice.

If you have a small amount of leftover chicken, meat, or fish, it can be added before the sauce—just long enough to heat through. If adding uncooked meats, add them after the onion. Cook them well before adding the raw vegetables.

Tofu is a nutritious addition to this dish. Cut it into small cubes and add just before serving—just long enough to allow the tofu to heat through.

Bread Pie

If you have nothing but stale bread in the freezer and a few eggs and cheese, you can make a hearty and filling meal. Break stale bread into small pieces, just bigger than a pea. For each cup of bread crumbs, add 1 egg, ¾ cup milk, ¼ cup grated cheese. Then use your imagination for seasonings. We like a dash or two of basil, cayenne pepper, and sage. Mix this all together and pour it into an oiled casserole dish. Bake at 350 degrees F until it sets and a toothpick inserted into the center comes out clean.

Southwestern Bread Pie

Follow the same recipe above and add a drained 6-ounce can of chopped chili peppers, a red bell pepper chopped finely for color. Omit the seasonings used for the plain bread pie. If you have frozen corn on hand, mix in ¼ cup for each cup of bread crumbs.

Other Combinations

There are hundreds of standby recipes—many probably already family favorites. The whole range of macaroni and other pasta dishes, simple egg and cheese dishes, quick soups and stews. Women's magazines and the food sections of newspapers weekly offer us new ideas.

The important thing is to THINK before you panic or call out to have Chinese food or pizza delivered! Look to see what two or three major ingredients you have. Thumb through the index of a cookbook to see what recipes use those ingredients. When you find a recipe with most (not necessarily all) of the ingredients which you have on hand, proceed.

It is also important to be brave! If the recipe calls for Dijon mustard and you have only Gulden's, either leave it out or try a dab of Gulden's. If a recipe says to use fresh marjoram and you do not even have marjoram leaves, only powdered marjoram—use it. Just use a little less.

The genius of famous chefs is in their ability to improvise—to make do (and to make fabulous) with what is available. You can too. Brave it!

COOKING IT RIGHT

Selecting low-fat, lean, and trim foods at the supermarket is certainly the first step to healthful eating and calorie control. But the leanest of ingredients can be sabotaged by your cooking method. Simple recipe changes can ensure that you do not add excess fat, sugar, and salt to undo your wise and economical choices.

Fats are the most dense and concentrated source of calories. A gram of pure protein or carbohydrate yields only 4 calories when burned. A gram of fat provides more than twice that amount. Fats are flavor carriers, so we commonly add fats to foods which otherwise are not all that fatty.

For example, we cook in butter, oils, lard, shortening, or margarine. We cover low-calorie vegetables with mayonnaise, dressings, sauces, and gravies which are high in fat. We spread butter and margarine on bread, noodles, potatoes, rice, and other foods which would otherwise be relatively low in calories.

Fats and Oils

To start cooking food right, we need to reduce the amount of fats and oils used in its preparation. If you serve meals weekly which contain fried foods, cut the number of fried-meal items to one or less per week. Serve the same foods prepared in some other manner. Instead of fried potatoes, serve boiled or baked potatoes (no sour cream! substitute a bit of grated cheese). Instead of frying fish, serve it poached, baked, or broiled with a dash of lemon juice.

Next reduce the amount of fats and oils used in recipes. In many main-dish items like casseroles, you can reduce the amount of fats by one-third or a half with no change in product quality. Omit butter, oil, or margarine when you boil noodles or pasta, cook rice, or boil vegetables.

Instead of fats or oils in the pan when sautéing vegetables or meats, use wine or broth or a nonstick vegetable-based spray.

Nonstick cooking sprays (in pump containers only—not in aerosol cans) contain very little fat and are virtually fat free.

The amount of fat called for in many baked goods can also be cut. In muffins, quick breads, and cookies, I cut the amount of butter, margarine, or oil called for to ⅔ the amount specified. If a cookie recipe calls for 1 cup of butter, I substitute ⅔ cup. I also do not bake cookies which are meant to be fatty such as butter cookies and shortbread.

It is not easy to cut the amount of fat in a cake recipe. Therefore, I do not make traditional cakes. Instead, when we want a cake, we have carrot, banana, date, or other nut breads. It is easy to reduce the fat in these recipes and still get an excellent dessert. Because the fruits add their own sweetness, I can also reduce the amount of sugar called for without minimizing the taste of the cake.

If you simply cannot live without a sauce or gravy, make one without fat. Add cold milk or fruit juice directly to flour or cornstarch (I find that the cornstarch works best) and blend until smooth. Then stir over medium heat until it thickens. Add herbs, spices, and lemon juice for flavor.

Dairy Products

Substituting low-fat dairy products for their fat cousins can save tons of calories. If a recipe calls for whole milk, substitute lowfat or skimmed. I substitute reconstituted nonfat milk because it also saves money.

If the recipe calls for heavy cream or half-and-half, substitute either evaporated whole or evaporated skimmed milk, undiluted. Again, evaporated milk is a staple in my cabinet. When unexpected guests arrive, I can always whip up a quiche using leftover vegetables and evaporated milk. You just follow a basic quiche recipe, substituting whole or skim evaporated milk for the cream or sour cream called for in the recipe.

Low-fat yogurt is a great substitute for sour cream in dips, sauces, and gravies. It has a slightly tarter flavor which may call for more seasonings to balance its bite. It also separates when used in cooked recipes. To overcome this, make a roux of cornstarch and yogurt and stir into the cooking sauce. It should smooth out.

Low-fat cottage cheese can replace ricotta in casseroles. My husband, who is Italian-American, does not notice the difference. I also make a "mock" egg salad filling for his sandwiches from low-fat cottage cheese with a bit of grated Cheddar cheese, turmeric, pepper, chopped celery, and onions.

TABLE 5.3 DAIRY PRODUCT SUBSTITUTIONS TO CUT CALORIES

Substitute	For	Calories Saved
1 cup 1% fat milk	1 cup whole milk	50
1 cup skim evaporated milk, undiluted	1 cup heavy cream	640
1 cup plain low-fat yogurt	1 cup sour cream	375
1 cup plain low-fat yogurt	1 cup regular mayonnaise	1455
1 cup blended low-fat cottage cheese	1 cup sour cream	305
1 cup low-fat cottage cheese	1 cup whole-milk ricotta cheese	250
1 cup regular cottage cheese	1 cup whole-milk ricotta cheese	190
1 cup part-skim ricotta cheese	1 cup whole-milk ricotta cheese	90
1 cup white sauce made with 1% fat milk, 2 tbsp flour, no fat	1 cup whole-milk white sauce made with 2 tbsp flour, and 2 tbsp butter	250
1 oz low-fat processed cheese	1 oz Cheddar cheese	60
¼ cup diet margarine	¼ cup regular margarine or butter	205
½ cup reduced-calorie mayonnaise	½ cup regular mayonnaise	480

Source: "Tufts University Diet and Nutrition Letter," Vol. 2, No. 7, September 1984.

Several low-fat margarines, mayonnaises, and salad dressings are available. Diet margarines have half the calories as regular margarine. They are made by whipping water into margarine. Do not attempt to bake with them. The water content makes them unsuitable for substitution in baked goods. Low-calorie salad dressings and mayonnaiselike products (usually called sandwich spread) contain almost half the number of calories as do their fat-filled counterparts.

Meat and Poultry

We have talked about buying only the leanest cuts of meat and trimming all visible fats from them and removing the skin from poultry. You can go one step further and simply use less meat and poultry in recipes. If you are making a casserole, stew, stir-fried dish, potpie, or soup, add more vegetables and carbohydrate foods and reduce the amount of meats used. This will cut costs and calories.

I substitute other ingredients for meat in many recipes which call for meat. For example, red kidney beans are used in place of meat in minestrone soup, lasagne, enchilada pie, and other Mexican dishes, "meat" loaf, and other combination casserole dishes. I use tofu to replace part of the cheese in dishes calling for cheese and for the fish or poultry called for in many stir-fry and Oriental dishes. If you want to retain the taste of meat, substitute beans or tofu for only a part of the meat. This will still drastically cut calories and fat.

Cholesterol

If you are watching cholesterol in addition to fats, review the list of cholesterol contents of foods in table 2.10, page 52. When recipes call for lard, shortening, or butter, substitute less saturated fats such as margarine and the oils, safflower, soybean, corn, and so forth. These are easy to substitute, even in pie-crusts. Because oils are liquid, they mix easily with ingredients and therefore less oil can be used. Many recipe books give substitution instructions.

When a recipe calls for whole eggs, instead use just whites. All the cholesterol in eggs is concentrated in the yolks. Two whites can be used in place of one whole egg. Save whole eggs for those rare days when you want to indulge at breakfast-time and really appreciate their taste.

Salt and Spices

Salt is another saboteur of good eating. While traveling in France I noticed that salt was used very sparingly, if at all, in cooking. Unlike Americans, who often salt their already salted food before they taste it, the French are cautious with the shaker. One chef explained that a touch of salt can enhance and heighten the flavors of foods. But a heavy hand can mask and cover the delicate nuances.

We have some control over the amount of salt we use, since one-fourth of the salt in our diet is added at our stove and at the table. Omit salt from your recipes. Other spices and herbs can bring out the flavor of foods and add their own distinct personality.

For example, carrots are naturally somewhat high in salt. No need to salt them further. Add a sprinkle of nutmeg to them to accentuate their natural sweetness. A dash of dill on zucchini adds zest to an otherwise plain vegetable. Paprika added to cheese sauce (cheese is processed with salt and contains large amounts) lends color and flavor. Lemon juice is a fresh and perky salt substitute commonly used in France after cooking vegetables to bring out their flavor.

If you have been shy of spices and herbs because of their cost, remember that a little goes a long way. According to the American Spice Trade Association, an ounce of pepper will season 1440 eggs! An ounce of oregano is enough for 432 slices of pizza. Half an ounce of basil will flavor 104 servings of chicken cacciatore. An ounce and a half of chili powder will make 34 generous bowls of chili. And a mere one and one-eighth ounces of cinnamon will spice 456 slices of apple pie.

Sugar

The final calorie culprit is sugar. You can cut from one-fourth to one-half from your recipes and still have sweet, tasty products. When I first began cutting sugar from my cookies, I went overboard. The result was a perfectly good-looking oatmeal cookie that, except for the pieces of dried dates, tasted like paste!

To start, cut one-third of the sugar called for. This works well in pie fillings, cookies, nut breads, puddings, fruit crisps, and molded desserts. A dash more vanilla or almond extract, cinnamon or nutmeg, will enhance the flavor without adding calories. Sugar contains about 200 calories per a quarter cup. Spices contain none.

When the recipe contains fruit, you can cut the sugar even further. The fruit will lend its own natural sweetness to the product. Notice products which are made for people who have diabetes. They use very little sugar and often do not use sugar substitutes. They are naturally sweetened with fruits and spices.

We do not eat desserts such as cakes, puddings, pies. On rare occasion, for a complicated and fanfare dinner, I will make a fruit tart. I use a standard whole wheat sugar cookie recipe for the crust with the sugar cut to half that called for. This is pressed into a fluted springform pan and baked. After it cools, I arrange fresh slices of fruit on top in an elaborate pattern. For a glaze, one tablespoon of jam (apricot) is diluted with water and heated, then spread over the fruit. This is a beautiful dessert which always gets rave reviews for its appearance and its fresh, juicy flavor.

Cutting back on fats, salt, and sugar does not mean cutting back on flavor. In the past several years, the great chefs of the West, from the late James Beard to Craig Claiborne to Julia Child, have all reduced these ingredients in their cooking. Several of them have published low-fat, low-sodium, and low-calorie cookbooks.

Nouvelle cuisine, a simple French cooking style which follows these same principles, has become the new standard for haute cuisine restaurants in New York and other major cities. Like traditional Japanese cooking, emphasis is placed upon delicate differences in flavor contrasted with breathtakingly beautiful presentation.

We have much to learn from these fashion leaders. Glamorous food is no longer cloaked in cream, smothered in sauce, or bubbling in butter. And glamorous people are no longer overweight. The new standard is lean and the new cooking is light on calories and distinct in flavor.

6. Purchasing Supplies for Home, Inc.

A major function of corporate management is the purchase and acquisition of supplies and goods to be used in product manufacturing. Translated, their job is to find the best buys possible within strict budgetary confines. Corporate profit margins are as much dependent on quality, low-cost inputs as they are on labor and other costs.

To ensure that best buys are found, corporations rely upon detailed specifications to describe exactly what they want, and an elaborate system of bids from suppliers who offer to sell it to them at varying prices. The corporation then picks the best price and best supplier for the services or goods needed.

Price is determined by the purpose of the goods, the amount needed, and the time of purchase. Paint to be used on the outside of a car must have different qualities from paint used on an inside engine part. Parts which are used frequently and in large number, like nuts and bolts, can be purchased in bulk. They can also be purchased when prices are good rather than on an as-needed basis since they are an input item which is always in demand.

These decisions are not unlike those you make in the kitchen. First, you have a somewhat fixed budget for food just as manufacturers do for their input items. Like manufacturers, there are certain items you use regularly which are part of a standard inventory. These are basic ingredients like flour, butter, beans, which you use in many recipes and which should always be on hand.

For each item you will need a supplier. The right supplier can offer you bargain savings and services.

And as purchasing officer, you must be alert to best buys for the purpose. Should you buy a Grade A or a Grade C peach to make peach cobbler? The choices you make can make or break the budget. They can determine whether you spend a moderate or excessive amount of the family funds on food.

DO DOLLARS STRETCH?

The cost of food is not going down. An average, middle-income family of four (two adults and two school-aged children) spent $47.10 weekly in September 1969, $94.50 weekly in July 1979, and $116.20 weekly in July 1984 for food. What is stretching is clearly not the dollar but rather our ability to make wise and economical food choices.

Hope for a downward turn of the price curve is about like wishing that some previously unknown rich uncle will leave you $1 million. Even presidents are no longer foolish enough to promise us a chicken in every pot when the cost of chicken has increased 23 percent in the past five years.

Level of income is not directly related to level of nutrition or wise buying. With so many food items to choose from (over 24,000 in the average grocery store), lack of time, little interest, inadequate nutritional knowledge, variations in food prices, and lack of a plan for purchases, it is easy to be a baffled buyer regardless of family income.

FUSS BUDGET

Random spending can squander the family's fortunes. If you do not already know, you should determine what your actual current costs are for housing, utilities, transportation, clothing, other fixed and recurring costs, and food. As a rule of thumb, your total food costs, both for meals eaten at home and those eaten away from home, should not exceed 18 percent of your family budget.

To find out what your weekly food costs are, save all of your grocery and food sales receipts for the next three months. Add them up. Subtract 20 percent of the total for nonfood items (the laundry soap, hair spray, and so forth). Add the amount for meals away from home during this same time period. Now divide by twelve (the number of weeks in three months).

For comparison, the U.S. Department of Agriculture publishes a quarterly estimate of the cost of food for a family of four (table 6.1). Their figures assume that all food is bought at the store and prepared at home. It does not include cost of meals away from home, alcoholic beverages, pet food, soap, cigarettes, paper goods, and other nonfood items commonly bought at the store.

TABLE 6.1 USDA WEEKLY COST OF FOOD AT HOME, JULY 1984

	Low-Cost	Moderate-Cost	Liberal
Families			
Family of 2 (20–50)	$45.90	$56.50	$69.60
Family of 2 (51 and over)	43.90	53.80	64.10
Family of 4 with preschoolers	65.90	80.40	98.10
Family of 4 with elementary-school children	77.60	96.90	116.20
Individuals in Four-Person Families			
Children			
1–2 years	11.50	13.40	16.10
3–5 years	12.70	15.60	18.70
6–8 years	16.80	21.00	24.50
9–11 years	19.10	24.50	28.40
Females			
12–19 years	18.80	22.60	27.30
20–50 years	19.50	23.60	29.90
51 and over	18.80	23.10	27.50
Males			
12–14 years	21.70	27.00	31.60
15–19 years	22.60	27.80	32.30
20–50 years	22.20	27.80	33.40
51 and over	21.10	25.80	30.80

If you spend about the same amount for food weekly as the cost-of-food plans, you will know that your spending is in line with other families of about the same size. If you spend a great deal less, you may not be providing the assortment of food your family actually needs.

If your costs exceed this, the following better buys guide may help you cut costs without cutting quality. You also need to consider changing family food practices. Altering food habits to fit a budget is not a new concept. A 1982 survey for *Woman's Day* magazine revealed that 49 percent (about 1 out of every 2) shoppers have made some changes in the food they eat and serve in the past few years. Their major motivation was not to improve diets but to fight inflation.

The menus beginning on page 112 and the best buys guides which follow on page 164 give cost-cutting tips while keeping quality and nutrition high. Corporations have accountants, financial planners and managers, and others who fuss with corporate budgets to ensure controlled spending. You will have to become the family fuss-budget.

INVENTORY MANAGEMENT

Manufacturers keep close control over their inventory of components required to produce the finished product. An assembly line cannot wait while the manager runs down to the store for more parts. To avoid the cost of delays, manufacturers use continuous inventories—often computerized systems—which automatically record items removed from stock and place orders to replace them. Kitchens in institutions, hotels, and restaurants use similar systems.

Manufacturers do not make purchases of goods which they do not have plans to use. Mr. Iacocca does not have a Jaguar carburetor in the warehouse just in case he decides to make a Jaguar. Neither does he buy twenty Volkswagen hubcaps because they are selling at a good price. These items have no place in his plans and are not in his inventory, tying up space and money.

A household food inventory should be equally tightly controlled. An ongoing list is needed to replace staples as they are used. A notepad near the cabinet or refrigerator to jot down items for restock as they are used will ensure that you are never without the basics.

Neither should there be money tied up in food goods that will not become part of meals. A $6 can of caviar that you bought two years ago is like a Jaguar carburetor in Mr. Iacocca's warehouse. So are the ten cans of corn that you bought at a good price, even though no one in your family is crazy about canned corn.

Stocking Staples

When pioneer women left for the frontiers, they left behind their bouquet garni, tarragon, and chervil. They took only those things which were essential and versatile, the simple staples around which they could build basic meals. Among these were flour, sugar, salt, coffee, beans.

Every household has a staples list—those foods which are purchased regularly and are the mainstays of the diet. Following are the best buys for nutritional quality, cost, and true versatility in each of the food groups used in menu planning. I actually have a checklist of staples posted in the kitchen so that we can check off items as they are used up and restock them.

Here is my list of nonperishable staples. These are items which can be stored. I purchase them when they are on sale and keep them until used. You can make your own checklist of those staples which you commonly use.

STAPLES: NONPERISHABLE

nonfat dry milk		canned milk		whole wheat flour	
baking powders and soda		cornmeal		tuna, water-packed	
wheat germ and bran		honey and molasses		pastas, several types	
rice		canned tomato paste		canned tomatoes and sauce	
beans, lentils, etc.		popcorn		canned clams	
oil: safflower and olive		vinegar: cider and wine		peanut butter	
spices and seasonings		raisins		sunflower seeds	
walnuts		almonds		bread crumbs	
oatmeal		cornstarch		soy sauce and tamari sauce	
sesame oil		sherry wine		unflavored gelatin	
olives		tea, coffee		extracts: vanilla, almond	

Generally you can save up to 6 percent when you purchase these items when they are in good supply and when they are featured as sale items. Again, make your own checklist of frequently used items.

(See Mother Hubbard's cupboard, page 145, for menus from a barren shelf.)

Before shopping, check weekly menus and recipes for items

STAPLES: PERISHABLE

fresh milk		potatoes		yogurt	
cottage cheese		juices		breads, at least two	
cheese		fresh vegetables		types for sandwiches	
frozen pastry shells		frozen spinach		fresh fruits	
frozen peas		tortillas		onions and garlic	

that will be needed for the week's meals. This will prevent a last-minute trip to the market to get a forgotten ingredient.

Check newspaper advertisements for specials. You may want to alter your menu plans if a particularly good buy is available. Don't buy specials unless they fit your menu plans or can be worked into them. Volkswagen hubcaps won't fit on Fords.

Also do not buy more than you can use or store. Ten pounds of potatoes which will rot before you can use them all is not a bargain. Neither is three gallons of ice cream if your family eats it all in one week and adds unnecessary calories to their intake.

No purchase should be made on impulse without a plan. This does not preclude purchasing staples or items for future use when they are a good price and they fit into your overall planning scheme. These should be basic, no-frill items, not Jaguar parts.

Impulse purchases can add hundreds of dollars per year to your grocery bill. Suppose you spend an extra $2.09 each week for a bag of chips or cookies. That is $108.68 per year. If you buy several unplanned items, the extras add up quickly.

LOCATING SUPPLIERS

Many types of grocers, produce markets, and specialty food stores exist today. How do you decide where to shop? The nearest grocer may not be the cheapest. Driving to several grocers in pursuit of "specials" may waste more time than it saves money. How do you decide?

Price

Obviously, the most important criterion is price. Take your staples list and compare prices among several grocers which you are considering. I shopped for almost one year at a market one block from my Manhattan apartment before realizing that by walking an additional half block to an alternate market, considerable savings on all my standard purchases were available.

Stores which list the price of the item and the price per unit on the shelf will help you compare prices. Also, make sure that individual items are marked with prices. Checkout clerks do not always remember prices.

Check specialty shop prices. The most acclaimed may not always be the most expensive for the quality. For example, in New York City, Zabar's, probably the world's most famous deli, offers cheeses regularly at prices substantially below those charged by supermarkets in the same neighborhood. Similarly, their special coffees are at least a dollar per pound cheaper than in regular groceries. Since the shop is out of my way, I buy enough coffee and cheese once monthly to last.

Bulk purchase or warehouse stores may provide substantial savings when you want to purchase staple items, such as dry and canned goods, in quantity. Some bulk purchase stores require you to bring your own containers to carry away your goods. Spices, flour, cereals, and so forth are offered in open bins and jars. You scoop out the amount you need.

Warehouses may sell by case or lot only. You can often buy goods at as little as 10 percent above wholesale costs. Be careful not to buy more than you can realistically use, nor to buy "VW hubcaps"!

Appearance and Service

Stores which are well-lighted, well-ventilated, and clean ensure that the food you purchase will be clean and safe from pest infestation.

Stores which have aisle labels or directories can save you time in locating items. Those with an excess of banners, posters, and aisle promotional displays may entice you to purchase items which are not needed. Store managers depend on a certain amount of impulse buying, encouraged by in-store advertising and end-aisle promotions, to increase their sales dollars.

Hours of operation may influence your choice. I like to shop early in the morning before midday shoppers crowd the aisles, or late at night after the dinner-hour rush subsides.

Check-cashing service is crucial for me. I rarely carry more than $20 in cash (for fear of being mugged!) and need to write a check for our groceries. Stores which give credit to their customers often charge more for their goods to compensate for losses when the credit customer fails to pay or pays in an untimely manner.

Delivery services are rare in urban communities but can be a boon to those without cars who live in inner cities. Check to see what the average delivery time is. If your groceries are left sitting for an hour, milk and other perishable items will become warm. Better to have family members help you carry groceries or invest in a shopping cart to carry things home yourself.

Also check to see what the charge is for delivery. Even if you have a car, you may on occasion want to call for a delivery of a forgotten menu item. You are balancing the value of your time against the cost of delivery. Delivery does add to the cost of your food.

Sanitation

Perishables, meat, dairy, and egg products should be refrigerated at a temperature of 42 degrees F or lower. Check to make sure that the display cases are kept clean with no dried milk, dried blood, broken eggs, etc.

Frozen foods should be frozen solid. Give the "squeeze the Charmin" test to ice-cream boxes. If they are soft, the freezers are not cold enough and other foods will be too warm too.

If produce is wilted, dry, dirty, tossed in the case haphazardly, and poorly trimmed, it is not a good buy. This area of a grocery requires considerable and constant attention. Notice whether there is a person in charge of the produce department who is present and caring for the fruits and vegetables.

"Buy-It-Fast" Stores

Convenience stores dot our cities and suburbs like freckles on a frog. Their convenience is based upon their hours of service—usually long before and after traditional markets close.

The range of foods which they offer is limited. Usually the only fresh items stocked are dairy products and eggs. Their primary sales are of canned goods, beer, snack items, magazines, aspirins, and other sundries.

Delicatessens offer "we-have-it-here-and-now" service. They

cater to workers on meal breaks who want a quick sandwich or snack and to party givers who want trays of cold cuts prepared. Limited selections of grocery items are often offered.

Because deli food is prepared and ready-to-eat, it has the cost of preparation built in and is more expensive than buying the ingredients to prepare the items at home. However, it may be less expensive than eating out on nights when you just don't feel like cooking. You can get a roasted chicken, a loaf of specialty bread, a three-bean salad, some fresh fruit, and milk, and you have a meal.

For me, the ideal market is one with a full range of grocery items, an expansive fresh produce section, a wine and cheese shop, and a deli. I then have to make only one stop and have to stand in a checkout line only once.

BETTER BUYS FOR THE BUCK

Price, quality, and appropriateness for your menu purposes are the key factors in food selection.

Unit Pricing

Most markets today list the price and the unit price (price per ounce, gram, pound, pint, quart, liter, etc.) on the shelf with the product to save you time in making comparisons. Generally the price of the container is in bold print and the price per unit is in small, lighter print, or actual statement of which price is the unit price is made.

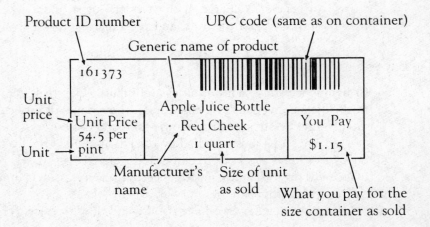

If unit prices are not listed, divide the total cost by the number of basic units (ounces, grams, pounds, pint, quart, liter, and so forth) then compare. For example, which is the best buy: the small size, Can A at 29 cents for 14 ounces, or the large size, Can B at 50 cents for 1 pound, 15 ounces?

$$\text{Can A: } \frac{29¢}{14 \text{ oz}} = 2.1¢ \text{ per oz}$$

$$\text{Can B: } \frac{50¢}{31 \text{ oz}} = 1.6¢ \text{ per oz}$$

Even though the larger size is less expensive, do not buy it if you can not use the larger quantity.

Items marked as "sale" and placed at the end of an aisle may not in fact be the least expensive. They may be a reduction in the normal price of that item or brand, but not necessarily the best buy. Calculate the unit price to be sure.

Also calculate the actual cost per unit in twofer sales. Two for 39 cents sounds like a bargain until you realize that individual units usually sell for 16 cents each. This twofer costs almost 4 cents more per unit.

The least expensive is not always equal quality and it is certainly not always worse quality. Select foods in a form which fits their intended use. Consider alternative forms (fresh, frozen, refrigerated, canned, dried) as well as brand, grade, quantity, size, and convenience. For example, Brand B peaches canned in natural juice are a better buy for making preserves or pies than fresh No. 1 peaches.

Quality and Appropriate Form

The year I was born there were only three kinds of vinegar: apple cider vinegar in white or brown and wine vinegar. Today you can buy vinegars made from every kind of fruit, from several different wines, and with a number of seasonings added to the bottle.

My parents bought coffee in a can with two options: regular or drip grind. Today we can buy coffees labeled by the type of roast, country in which it was grown, added flavors from almond to cinnamon, chocolate, and orange peel, with or without caffeine, in various grinds, and several instant forms.

It is no wonder that choosing is one of the greatest challenges when purchasing foods. Add the desire to get the most nutrition at the best price and choice is even more complicated.

Following is a compendium of staple food items with tips on how to read labels, compare quality, select the form most appropriate for your uses, and cut costs while maximizing nutrient content. The buying tips are grouped by the food groups used in menu planning.

FRUIT AND VEGETABLE GROUPS

Juices

It is no easy task to find a needle in a haystack nor to know whether there is real fruit juice in what looks like fruit juice. Manufacturers have mixed fruit flavors, sugars, and real juice into a myriad of drinks and beverages with names and pictures on the label suggesting that it contains the real stuff. You have to read the label to know for sure.

If the label says "juice" then it is "juice." You will, of course, feel reassured if it says "pure" or "100%" but it may not always. If the label says "drink," "cocktail," "ade," "punch," or any other juicy-sounding name, it is not pure, 100 percent fruit juice. It is some combination of water, sugar, citric acid, flavorings, and possibly some fruit juice.

Some containers today will state the percentage of fruit juice on the label—10 percent real fruit juice or 35 percent pure juice. But usually they don't. Ades are not required to have any more than 25 percent juice and can have less. Drinks or punches may have only 10 percent or some as low as 3 percent. Read the ingredients label to see what is in the container. Do not pay fruit juice prices for sugared, flavored water.

Real Orange Juice

Homemade, fresh-squeezed orange juice is the most expensive. It is also time consuming to prepare—even when you have an electric juicer. Many markets today have machines which squeeze the juice before your eyes and put it in cartons or bottles for sale. This too is expensive.

Orange juice in a carton or bottle in the dairy case is usually the same juice that you could make yourself at home with frozen concentrate. Look for the word "reconstituted" which means that it is not fresh squeezed. It costs more if the bottler adds the water than if you do.

The two best buys are frozen concentrate, which tastes most like fresh juice when reconstituted, and canned juice. Nationally advertised brand-name frozen concentrate is more expensive than the grocery store's own brand or generic (no-name) labels.

Buy straight juice. Several manufacturers add pulp and peel to their product to make it look more like fresh squeezed. Generally they also add sugar. If you want the pulp, read the label to make sure that nothing else is added.

In terms of vitamin C content, fresh does contain slightly more than juice made from frozen concentrate. And juice made from frozen concentrate contains slightly more C than canned juice.

Soft Drinks and Substitutes

For some reason, we have gotten out of the habit of drinking water and instead often turn to sweetened beverages to quench our thirst. Soft drinks are a nutritional and economic waste. They contain no nutrients and are essentially expensive, flavored, sugared water.

Our soft drink habit is also a cost to the earth. Even though some states have can return programs, we still use a good share of our earth's metal resources to produce cans which are not recycled. The pop-tops and caps from our beverage cans and bottles pollute streets and streams. This is no small problem. We annually throw away more than 60 billion cans and bottles.

In this same category of nutritionally wasteful beverages falls drink mixes, punches, and ades (table 6.2). They are an expensive form in which to buy sugar.

TABLE 6.2 JUICE SUBSTITUTE BEVERAGES COMPARED

12-Ounce Serving	Tsp Sugar	% Fruit Juice	Calories	Cost
Orange soda	11.8	0	188	37¢
Kool-Aid	8.2–9	0	131–144	9¢
Hawaiian Punch	9.7	0	156	17¢
Tang	11.4	0	182	12¢
Cranberry juice cocktail	9.6	27	205	50¢
Sugar	1	0	16	0.004¢

Source: Adapted from "Nutrition Action," October 1984, with permission from the Center for Science in the Public Interest, Washington, D.C.

Instead, have your kids mix their own "fruit soda" using real fruit juices. It saves money and calories and adds important vitamins and minerals (table 6.3).

TABLE 6.3 SODA vs. FIZZLE

Orange Soda	Orange Fizzle
10 oz carbonated water	½ cup carbonated water
3 tbsp sugar	¾ cup orange juice
Several drops artificial orange color and flavoring	
Caffeine (optional)	
Cost: 26¢	Cost: 24¢
Sugar: sucrose (sugar) added	Sugar: natural fruit sugar, no sugar added
Calories: 150	Calories: 90
Color and flavoring: all artificial	Color and flavoring: natural
Nutrients: none except calories	Nutrients: vitamin C, vitamin A, folic acid potassium

Fresh Produce

Improvements in harvesting methods, packaging, transportation, and storage have extended the traditional season in which fresh produce is available almost year round. There are still peak harvest seasons when fresh goods are most plentiful and their prices are best. Fresh produce is also at its best in flavor and nutrition during this time.

Where to Get It

The best buys are locally grown produce. They are fresher and you do not pay packing and shipping costs. If you are planning to make and freeze large numbers of fruit pies or to can jams or freeze vegetables yourself, you can sometimes go directly to the fields to pick them. The savings are considerable, but this can only be done if you have time.

When I lived in Washington, D.C., my friends and I drove to Virginia each fall to pick baskets of apples. We would choose a pretty day and make it a picnic outing. In the evening we invited other friends to help peel, core, and prepare the apples for applesauce and apple pies. Each helper's reward was a slice of hot steaming pie to eat when the job was done and one frozen pie to take home.

The agriculture agent at your local Agriculture Extension Services (listed under county offices in the telephone directory) usually has a list of farmers who allow you to pick your own. They also may have lists of produce stands selling directly from field to you.

Produce terminals in many large cities and some small towns offer great bargains. Generally these are warehouse areas with stalls, loading docks, and other services provided for farmers to pull their trucks in and sell directly to bulk purchasers like restaurateurs and grocers.

These markets typically open before 4:00 A.M. and have completed their day's work by noon. While their primary service is offered to bulk buyers, individuals can usually make purchases. You must get there early or the best buys are gone. Professional chefs and buyers and specialty shop owners will be there early to choose top grades at bottom prices. If you wait until noon, you may find only culls. You may have to purchase in bulk boxes and containers. If so, ask a few neighbors to join you in buying and splitting the goods.

My first trip to a produce terminal was to the San Francisco Terminal Market as an undergraduate in dietetics at the University of California, Berkeley. I was so enamored with the smells, colors, hussle and bustle of the market, and orders being yelled in Italian and Chinese, that I totally neglected my assignment!

Many cities now sponsor farmers' markets or direct marketing locations where smaller truck crop farmers can bring pickups full of produce to sell in small-lot sizes to individual buyers. Washington, D.C.'s Eastern Market, Baltimore's Lexington Market, and New Orleans French Market are famous for their open-air farmers' market.

Grades

The U.S. Department of Agriculture sets standards for grading fresh produce. There is no requirement that the grades be used. However, if they are, then the product must meet the grade label given it. Generally these grades are used as a basis for trading between growers, shippers, wholesalers, and retailers rather than for consumer information. However, we do see the grade marking, sometimes on packages of carrots or onions, and sometimes in the grocer's advertisements.

The top vegetable grade is U.S. No. 1 or U.S. Fancy. Grades for fresh fruits are U.S. Fancy and U.S. No. 1 through No. 3. The quality of most fresh produce can be judged reasonably well by external appearance, without the help of a grade mark or other identification of quality. Some thumbnail hints which will help you find the best are:

1. Check for freshness—bright, lively color and crispness; no discoloration, no slimy or slick spots or white mold; no off odor.
2. Buy in season—quality is highest, freshness at a peak, prices more reasonable (see Seasonal Produce chart on page 172–73).
3. Shop for plentiful produce—watch newspaper and television ads to see what is in abundant supply. Prices are lowest when there is lots in the market. Strawberries can be as low as 59 cents a basket during season and as high as $2.59 a basket out of season.
4. Buy only what you will use—do not buy a cellobag of 2 dozen soft plums if your family will only eat 6–7 per week. The extras may spoil.
5. Handle all fresh produce with care—do not pinch, poke, or abuse! No molestia!
6. Buy it ripe—you can tell it is ripe if it smells like you want it to taste when you eat it.
   • If it is not ripe, store at room temperature for several days in a bowl or lightly opened paper bag. Do not store in sun; it will shrivel, sunburn, and rot.
   • If it is ripe, refrigerate in the produce bin of the refrigerator. Do not store near the freezer. Celery, lettuce, and other watery vegetables will become limp and wilted; fruits will bruise and lose their texture. Store potatoes, beets, and other root vegetables and onions in a cool dry closet or shelf . . . like the old root cellar!

Don't get carried away with picture-perfect produce. If you are going to slice and dice it for a fresh fruit salad, you can buy blemished or less than perfectly shaped fruit—usually at considerable savings. If you are going to make preserves or pies, then again, appearance in the whole form is not important.

Penny Foolish Snacks vs. Fruits:

For the same cost you can buy:

16 ounces of   OR   1 pound carrots
potato chips   plus 2 cucumbers
                            plus 2 green peppers
                            plus 2 zucchini

Nutrient comparison per serving:
PC = 1 oz. potato chips
V   = 1 large raw carrot

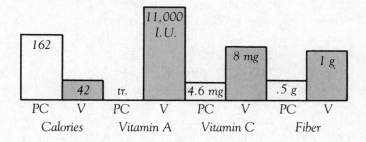

For the same cost you can buy:

19 ounces of   OR   ³/4 pound peaches
assorted cookies   plus 1 cantaloupe
                            plus 3 plums
                            plus ¹/2 pound grapes
                            plus 2 pears

Nutrient comparison per serving:
C = 1 chocolate cookie
F = ¹/4 of 5″ diameter cantaloupe

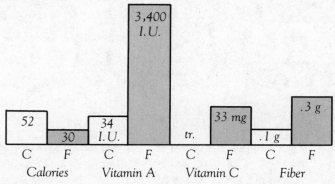

Penny Foolish Snacks vs. Fruits

Fresh fruits and vegetables are an economical and nutritious snack food. See charts (page 169) for what you can buy instead for the same cost.

Prices are lowest when fresh produce is in season and in abundant supply. The chart on pages 172–73 lists peak seasons for many fruits and vegetables.

Canned and Frozen Produce

The U.S. Department of Agriculture's Food Safety and Quality Service sets grade standards for canned and frozen produce. Here the grades are uniform between fruits and vegetables.

U.S. Grade A are the best. They are selected for excellent color, uniform size, weight, and shape, ripeness or tenderness, and freedom from blemishes. These are the sweetest fruits and most succulent, flavorful vegetables. U.S. Grade B are slightly less perfect than Grade A in color, uniformity, and texture. They are usually more mature and less tender or sweet.

U.S. Grade C vegetables are not so uniform in color and flavor and are usually more mature and less tender. They are a good buy for use in soups and stews. Grade C fruits may contain some broken and uneven pieces, and are less perfect in color and texture. These are also a good buy for use as an ingredient in other dishes.

U.S. grade appears in a shield-shaped marking on the container, as shown below.

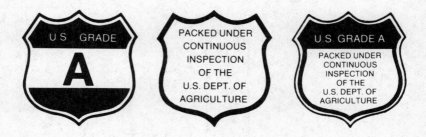

Many people believe that in-store brands (for example, those which are not nationally advertised like DelMonte and Libby's) and generic brands (those white labels with no-frills print) are lower-grade products. Sometimes they are but usually they are not. They are less expensive because their costs do not include fancy designer labels and paying Bill Cosby to visit your home via TV to convince you to buy the products.

Read the label to find the U.S. grade. The same product quality is often available at considerable savings in the store's own brand or in generic packaging.

TABLE 6.4 COST OF PEAS

Canned Peas (1 lb)	Description on Label	Cost in Cents
Generic[a]		47
Krasdale[b]	Tender Fancy	59
Libby's[c]	Sweet	69
DelMonte	Regular	69
DelMonte	No Salt Added	69
Green Giant	Very Young Tender	69
Le Sueur	Very Young Small	89
S & W	Fancy Early June	99

Source: New York City prices, November 1984.
[a]No frills, no name, brandless.
[b]Krasdale is store's own brand at Sloan's in New York.
[c]All of Libby's vegetables are salt-free.

There is no significant nutritional difference in these products. Where difference does occur is between forms: fresh, canned, or frozen. Fresh has the highest all-round quality—assuming that you do not cook it to death and leach out all the nutrients before eating it.

If purchased in season when supplies are abundant, fresh will be the best buy. When not in season, frozen may be the best buy. For a May dinner, I prepared Brussels sprouts and carrots. Brussels sprouts are not in season in May and the fresh ones were $1.39 per basket of 12 ounces. Frozen ones were 69 cents for 10 ounces. The texture, color, and flavor of the frozen did not perfectly match that of fresh, but the slightly lesser quality was worth the dramatic savings.

We find 10-ounce boxes of frozen vegetables to be too small for our needs. Four 2½-ounce servings are less vegetables than we eat. So when I do buy frozen vegetables, I buy them in plastic bags. They are generally several cents cheaper per ounce as well.

Canned produce has two potential nutritional drawbacks,

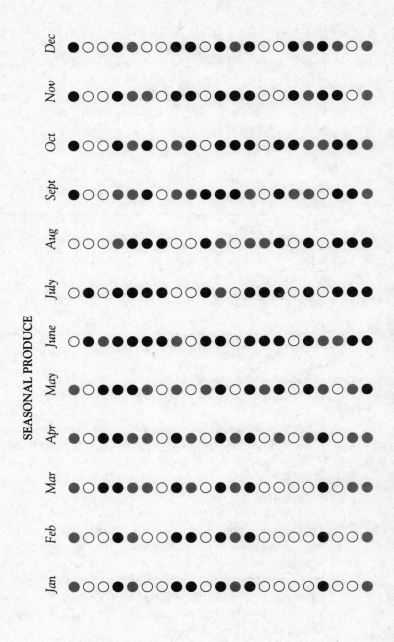

SEASONAL PRODUCE

Jan Feb Mar Apr May June July Aug Sept Oct Nov Dec

Lettuce
Limes
Mushrooms
Nectarines
Onions, dry
Oranges
Peaches
Pears
Peas
Peppers
Pineapples
Plums
Potatoes
Pumpkins
Radishes
Spinach
Squash
Strawberries
Sweet potatoes
Tomatoes
Watermelon

○ low supply to none available   ● fair supply   ● peak to good supply
Source: Courtesy of United Fresh Fruit and Vegetable Association.

both of which can be avoided. Canned fruits were traditionally canned in heavy syrups. This added significantly to the total calories in the form of simple sugar. Canned vegetables often have added salt.

Over the years nutritionists have advised people who use canned fruits, particularly during the winter when fresh produce was not available, to rinse off the syrup before eating. Today canners pack fruits in a choice of light syrup, natural fruit juices, or water. The calorie differences are striking (table 6.5). And so is the flavor. The light, natural, and water-packed fruits taste much more like fresh fruits than fruits canned in heavy syrup.

TABLE 6.5 COST OF PEACHES

Peach Slices (1 lb)	Tsp Added Sugar Per Serving	Calories Per Serving	Cost in Cents
Fresh raw	0	38	89
Packed in natural fruit juice	0	50	79
Packed in light syrup	0.8	50	79
Packed in heavy syrup	2.6	80	75
Packed in extra heavy syrup	3	85	75

Source: New York City prices, November 1984.
Note: The fresh peaches are at off-season prices, the highest.

Calories notwithstanding, some people just do not like the taste of canned fruit unless it is dripping in heavy syrup. An elderly arthritic patient I was seeing to reduce the weight on her painful joints, could not understand how anyone could eat water- or light-syrup-packed fruits. She loved fresh fruit. But canned fruit was just not canned fruit unless the liquid was sticky and thick. We gradually retrained her tastebuds. She admits that occasionally she must still have a peach half with all the golden, viscous, sugary fluid that she can scoop up with her spoon.

Our children are being raised at a time when fresh produce is available for a major part of the year from around the nation and from our southern neighbors in Mexico. We are far less dependent on canned fruits.

Canned and frozen vegetables have the hazards of added salt or sodium. Again, for years nutritionists told people to pour the salt brine from the can and add clear water for heating. We did this at the risk of washing away nutrients which had leached out into the canning fluid, but felt that the slight nutrient losses were less harmful than the added salt.

Manufacturers today offer an alternative. In 1982 two of the major vegetable processors, DelMonte and Libby's, introduced no-salt added canned vegetables. Almost everyone else in the industry has followed suit, offering no-salt or low-salt products. In most cases, they are offered at no added cost.

Frozen vegetables are often chilled to prefreezing temperature during processing, by soaking in a saltwater solution. This solution is drained off, but some salt may adhere. Read the label to see whether trace amounts of sodium or salt are mentioned. For most of us the amount is not significant. For those on a strict sodium-controlled diet, it might be (see table 6.6).

TABLE 6.6 SODIUM CONTENT OF CARROTS

Carrots (1 lb)	Sodium
Fresh, raw	175
Libby's no salt added[a]	175
DelMonte's no salt added	175
DelMonte's regular	1,070

[a]Libby's no longer even makes a salted version. Its entire line is no-salt.

Canned goods labeled "dietetic" or "diabetic" are available in many grocery stores and in most health food stores. Until the last few years, they were the only source for no-sugar/no-salt added foods. Today they have many competitors on the regular shelves of the store. There is no need to buy these higher-priced items—unless your dietitian has told you to do so, or you need the smaller serving size containers in which they are packed.

Sauces, Seasonings, Gravies

Both canned and frozen vegetables today are offered in a variety of sauces, seasonings, gravies, and combinations. Butter or cream sauces and gravies add variety to meals without adding extra work. The negative trade-off is that they also add extra calories, extra salt, and extra cost.

You are penny- and pound-wiser to purchase plain vegetables and add your own seasonings and to stir up your own "international fare" combinations. Omit the sauces, butter, and margarine when making your own. It saves calories, time, and cost.

DAIRY FOODS GROUP

Milk Products

When I was small, we drank so much milk that it was cheaper to keep a cow than to pay for milk deliveries. None of Bessie's milk (original name!) went to waste. What we couldn't drink, my mother's five younger brothers could.

Preparing the milk for drinking required strict sanitation. My grandmother would wash milk buckets thoroughly then bring the milk to scalding hot to kill all bacteria and germs. One of the worst burns I ever had in my life occurred in her kitchen. Milk buckets turned upside down on the kitchen floor to drain were perfect seats for me at three to sit on to watch my grandmother work. She had set a bucket of boiling milk on the floor to cool, when I waddled in to watch her. Without looking, I backed up to position myself in my favorite watching place, only to be greeted by searing pain. It took days for the blisters on my bottom to heal!

The process of applying heat to sterilize milk is called pasteurization. Raw, unsterilized milk can be purchased. The risks of contamination are high. If you are going to buy fresh dairy milk or commercial raw milk, two rules are critical: first, purchase raw milk only from certified dairies where cows are inspected regularly for disease and where sanitation practices are extremely cautious. Second, handle the milk with strict sanitation at home and use it within two days of purchase.

Imitation milk and milk products enjoyed a short vogue and are still available. These products contain milk which has had the milk fat removed. It has been replaced with a vegetable fat, most often palm or coconut oil. Both of these oils are higher in saturated fat than butter fat and therefore pose a greater risk of increasing your blood cholesterol levels than do natural milk products.

The popularity of the imitations resulted from their lower cost and the false belief that since they did not contain butter fat, they were healthier. To counter this impression, several regional dairy groups have started campaigns emphasizing the benefits of buying REAL milk products.

My opinion is that dairymen are right. Avoid imitation dairy products. Instead, purchase real milk products that are low-fat. All dairy products are now available in whole and low-fat forms:

milk, yogurt, cottage cheese, many cheeses. The calorie and cost savings can be significant when you buy low-fat or skim milk products (table 6.7).

TABLE 6.7 COST AND CALORIE CONTENT OF DAIRY FOODS

Dairy Item	Total Calories	% Calories From Fat	Cost
Whole milk	295	49	$0.99/half gallon
Low-fat milk	268	31	$1.07/half gallon
Skim milk	163	0.03	$0.95/half gallon
Cottage cheese	481	36	$1.19/16 oz
Low-fat cottage cheese	390	0.03	$1.29/16 oz
Yogurt	281	49	$1.59/32 oz
Low-fat yogurt	227	31	$1.59/32 oz

Source: Prices from Ridgewood, New Jersey, November 1984.

The only thing removed from low-fat dairy products is the fat. They still contain the same amount of protein, calcium, vitamins A and D, and other essential nutrients which make them an important food ingredient in our daily diets.

Chocolate and other flavored milks are favorites with children. When purchasing them, be sure to buy "milk" not "drink." The flavored drinks contain some milk but are not really full dairy products. You may pay the same or slightly less for the drink but you do not get your money's worth of nutrition (table 6.8). Drinks contain more fat and sugar than the real milk product. The fats which they contain may also be more saturated than the fats occurring naturally in milk. Coconut, cottonseed and palm oil are often added to these drinks.

TABLE 6.8 CHOCOLATE AND OTHER FLAVORED MILKS

	Protein gms	Fat gms	Carbohydrate gms	Calories	Cost ¢
Chocolate milk	8	5	26	179	65
Chocolate-flavored drink	5	11	36	260	63
Strawberry-flavored drink	8	10	36	270	55

Dried powdered and canned milks can add nutrition to your soups, sauces, and baked goods. I keep both types on hand just for this purpose. When making pancakes and cookies, I add an extra ½ to 1 cup of dry milk powders, some bran, and wheat germ to push up the nutritional value.

Yogurt

Yogurt, unknown to most Americans ten years ago, has become a best-selling dairy product. It has also become the victim of added sugar, flavoring, and coloring agents. Several yogurts marketed are more like dessert products than milk products.

Yogurt is a cultured milk product. That is, after milk has been pasteurized to kill all bacteria, active, live yeast cultures are added to it and it is kept warm for several hours. The yeast digests some of the milk sugar, causing fermentation, and forming a custardlike product.

Notwithstanding jokes about whether yogurt has more active culture than California, I personally prefer those yogurts in which the yeast is still alive. However, there is no significant nutritional difference between yogurts with live or those with attenuated (dead) yeast.

The best nutritional buy is plain yogurt. Add your own fruits or even whole fruit jams or preserves at home. This will cut cost and calories. A cup of flavored yogurt can contain as much as 280 calories. A cup of plain yogurt contains only 110. With fresh fruit added at home, the calories run up to less than 175.

A small number of people have an allergy to the lactose (sugar) that occurs naturally in milk. Because the yeast eats most of this sugar, people who are allergic can often eat yogurt and other cultured milk products, such as kefir, without any reaction.

I make most of the yogurt which we eat. It takes little time and Jennifer is fascinated by the process taking place. We do not use a fancy yogurt maker but make it in a large jar. Simply select a jar with a tight-fitting lid. Boil enough skim milk to almost fill the jar. Add ½ cup of powdered nonfat dry milk per 2 cups of milk. Mix and cool the milk to lukewarm. Add a heaping tablespoon of plain yogurt with live culture and mix. Wrap the jar in a dish towel and place it in a dark warm oven (mine has a pilot light which keeps it at about 85–90 degrees F). In 8 hours or so you will have fresh, homemade yogurt. It is ready when it thickens. Place it in the refrigerator until you are ready to use it.

Butter vs. Margarine

Butter is made by churning pasteurized cream. As a child, I thought that it was magic food. I would watch my grandmother as she poured cream into her churn, sat in her rocker, and whistled while she churned. About midway through her third lullaby, the butter "came" and separated from the cream. I was sure that it was the magic of her whistle that made it come.

Butter must be at least 80 percent milk fat by federal law. Salt and coloring may be added. Unsalted butter or sweet butter is often served in fancy restaurants. It has a deliciously delicate flavor which many prefer over salted.

Because of the high level of saturated fat in butter, it is solid at refrigerator temperatures and cannot be spread easily. Whipped butter spreads easily. It simply has air beaten in which makes it softer. The whipped-in air also cuts the calories down a bit. If like me, you love the taste of butter, you may want to use the whipped ones to keep fat and calories to a minimum.

Margarines are "imitation" butter made from various vegetable oils. Their initial popularity stemmed from their lower cost. Today they are lauded as a substitute for butter because of their reduced content of saturated fats and cholesterol.

Read the ingredient label when purchasing margarine. Many of the cheaper margarines are made with coconut and palm oil which are less expensive oils. They are also more saturated than butter fat. It would be better to eat butter than to use these margarines if you want to cut cholesterol.

The lowest-saturated-fat margarines are made with safflower, corn, or soybean oil which are polyunsaturated. You may pay more but they are the best nutritional buys.

However, remember that butter and margarine contain the same number of calories per serving. Using margarine cuts down on saturated fats but does not cut calories. Use both very sparingly.

Cheese

Cheese has been made for thousands of years from the milk of cows as well as goats, camels, asses, mares, buffaloes, and reindeer. We most commonly eat cow's milk cheeses.

Most cheese is "natural," that is, it is made directly from milk which has been curdled or coagulated and pressed to remove the liquid, then stored for various time periods to allow the bacteria or mold to ripen it.

Processed cheese is made from a blend or combination of one or more kinds of natural cheeses, an emulsifying agent, acids such as lactic or acetic, salt, and flavorings. The mixture is heated, which kills all bacteria. This cheese will store longer than natural cheeses, but in my opinion, it is higher in salt and lower in flavor than natural cheeses.

Processed cheese spreads come in jars and tubes. They have a higher moisture content, to make them spreadable, and thereby have a diluted protein content.

Imitation cheese products are found in some markets. Like imitation milk, their butterfat has been replaced by some other (usually less expensive) fat.

Generally, the price of cheese increases with the time required to age it. Mold-ripened cheeses are more difficult to make and are more expensive than bacteria-ripened cheeses.

The amount of fat in a cheese determines the degree of softness. The higher the fat, the softer the cheese. For those who are watching their intake of dietary fat and cholesterol, it would be wise to limit the amount of cheese eaten and to give preference to the hard cheeses.

Many of my patients believe that cheese is fattening. A 1-ounce cube of cheese contains no more calories than a small Danish or a 1-ounce chocolate. What seems to be the problem is that cheese is an easy-to-grab snack food. If you are watching your weight, do include cheese in your diets (table 6.9). It is an excellent source of protein and calcium. But keep the amount in control or you will soon look like a wheel of Brie.

Tofu

Another product found in the dairy case which can be used like cheese or cottage cheese is tofu. Also called bean curd, it is a pale white, bland-tasting, cheeselike product made from fermented soybeans. It is cut into squares and sold in a water pack. It is not a dairy product and is sometimes sold in the fresh-produce section of the store.

For over 2000 years, tofu has been one of the primary sources of protein for Asians. It is rapidly becoming popular in the West due to its good protein and calcium content, low cost, and versatility.

TABLE 6.9 NATURAL CHEESE

Unripened		Soft Ripened	
Soft	Semisoft	Mold	Bacteria
Baker's	Gjetost	Brie	Limburger
Cottage	Mozzarella	Camembert	Liederkranz
Cream	Mysost		
Neufchâtel			
Pot			
Riccota			
Teleme			

Semisoft Ripened		Firm Ripened	Hard
Mold	Bacteria	Bacteria	Bacteria
Blue	Bel Paese	Cheddar	Cheshire
Gorgonzola	Brick	Colby	Parmesan
Roquefort	Fontina	Edam	Romano
Stilton	Gouda	Emmenthaler	Sapsago
	Monterey	Gruyère	
	Muenster	Kumminost	
	Port du	Nokkelost	
	Salut	Provolone	
	Tilsit	Swiss	
	Trappist		

Source: From USDA, *How to Buy Cheese*, May 1977.

It is fat free and low in calories. In addition to the many stir-fried and Oriental dishes in which it is used, it can be added to favorite home recipes including soups, spreads, dips, salads, sauces, sandwiches, and casseroles. I put it in lasagna to replace part of the cheese.

A manufacturer has recently introduced a frozen dessert called Tofutti which is made from tofu. Unlike ice cream, it is fat-free, and is lower in sugar content than frozen yogurt or ice cream. It promises to be the "dessert" of the fitness generation.

CARBOHYDRATE FOODS GROUP

Whole Grain Foods

Whole grains such as barley, bulgur, millet, wheat berries were once part of our meals. They were served as a side dish like rice or potatoes or in soups and gruels. Few of us any longer use these grains, although couscous (a Middle Eastern grain) and bulgur in a dish called tabooli have enjoyed some vogue. Most of the grain products which we eat today have been processed into breads and cereals.

Bread, cereal, and grain products are among the complex carbohydrate foods which we are today encouraging consumers to eat more of. Whole grain foods are good sources of the B-vitamin complex, several trace minerals, and of fiber.

The form in which they are eaten is important. Grain-based products such as cakes, cookies, many crackers, and snack foods have proportionally more fat and sugar than grain. Emphasis should be put on selecting products such as whole grain breads and cereals and pasta products which have a minimum of fat and sugar added.

Whole grain products are made from the whole kernel of wheat and contain the bran as well as the germ. Most of the nutrients in wheat are concentrated in the kernel. Whole grain products will have more minerals, vitamins, slightly more protein and fiber than products made from refined white flours.

By law, most refined white flours are enriched. That is, some of the nutrients which were removed during the milling process are added back to the flour. Thiamine, riboflavin, niacin, and iron are added back to the same level as the whole grain product contains. However, several other nutrients (magnesium, calcium, potassium, phosphorus, manganese, molybdenum, vitamin B-6, pantothenic acid, and vitamin E) are partially lost during milling and are not added by enrichment. It is true that these nutrients occur only in very small amounts in grains. There also are other food sources of them in our diets. Nonetheless, I still prefer to have all the things God originally put in my food still present when I eat it.

Breads

Do not be misled by labels. If the product contains the whole grain it should say "whole grain" or "whole wheat," or "100% rye flour" on the label. Words such as "wheat bread" or "natural" or "full-grain" do not guarantee that the whole grain kernel has been used.

Color is also not an indicator of whether the product is whole grain. Many breads and cereals have coloring added to make them look more like "old-fashioned rye or pumpernickel" or "whole wheat."

Use a wide variety of breads in family meals. This will allow everyone's favorite to be included and will ensure access to the full range of nutrients available from breads. Day-old breads are no less nutritious than baked-today breads. I freeze all bread anyway, so it is always at least a day old.

Very few people make their own breads today. While as much as 60 percent of the cost of bread can be saved, it takes time. If you do decide to make bread, or if your teenagers do, make four or five loaves at a time. You can freeze the extras. This is more efficient than making one or two loaves at a time.

I do not make yeast breads regularly but I do make fruit breads for use at breakfast. Banana, raisin, cranberry, dried apricot, and apple breads are breakfast favorites. These take very little time to make in my food processor. I make two and freeze them. We cut off just enough for breakfast and heat it in the toaster oven. I also make whole wheat bran muffins for breakfast, lunches, and snacks. These too are frozen.

Pastas

There are more than one hundred varieties of pastas. We are most familiar with spaghetti, macaroni, lasagne, and flat noodles. Pastas exist in a multitude of shapes from spirals to corkscrews to bows to shells to ribbons to angel hair. They come in plain wheat and in combination varieties, including artichoke, beet, carrot, parsley, tomato, and spinach, which lend beautiful colors.

Pasta became popular when long-distance runners began to hail it as an excellent before-marathon food. It can make simple, quick, inexpensive, and nourishing family meals. My husband, who is Italian-American, has introduced me to all the varieties. We use pasta as a main dish at least as frequently as we do as a side dish.

There are no significant nutritional differences between imported and domestic varieties of pasta. All are made from semolina flour, a high gluten flour made from durum wheat. Fresh pastas, sold in the deli department or refrigerator section of the grocery, are considerably more expensive than either imported or domestic dry pastas.

I am no judge of their quality. A close friend who manufactures and imports pastas from Italy swears that fresh pastas are made of lower-grade flours than dried ones and that the quality of the product is inferior. You can decide for yourself. In terms of straight cost, the dried pastas are a better buy. They also give you the option to store them for future meals.

Crackers

Crackers made from various grains are a popular snack food. Since they are not cookies, we often allow ourselves to indulge, thinking that we are saving calories. Many of them contain so much fat that they contain more calories than the cheese we spread on top of them or the cookies we avoided when we ate them. You can get an idea of how high in fat a cracker is by looking for a greasy spot. If the cracker leaves smudges on a napkin, it's greasy. Wheat Thins, Triscuits, Ritz, and many assorted variety crackers have as much as 40–50 percent of their calories as fat (table 6.10). If you are using these crackers to transport cream cheese, cheese spreads, and other snack dips to your lips, you are doubling trouble.

There are low-fat crackers on the shelf. Ry Krisp, Wasa rye crackers, Finn Crisps, pretzels, and rice cakes contain very little fat. Read the labels to see what is in the product. If there is a nutrition label, check the number of calories per cracker. You could be shocked to learn that so many calories could come in such an innocent-looking little square.

TABLE 6.10 CALORIES IN CRACKERS

Cracker (approx. 1 oz)	Calories	Fat (g)
Ritz	150	8
Wheat Thins	140	6
Triscuits	140	5
Ry Krisp	100	0

Finally, note the cost. Pound for pound, crackers are costly. Think carefully about how they are to be used in family nutrition and whether another grain product might do the job just as well. For example, peanut butter snacks for children can be put on toast points as easily as on crackers. Party hors d'oeuvres can also be spread on bread. You will save cost and calories.

Cereals

Numerous nutrition advocates claim that many of our popular breakfast cereals should be sold from the candy counter and not the cereal shelf. There is good reason for the claim. Some children's cereals contain as much as 30–50 percent sugar.

Avoid these cereals. Read the label. If sugar or sugar by any of its other names (see page 30) appears as the first or one of the first three ingredients, do not buy the cereal. Remember, sugar costs only 44 cents per pound. Why pay $1.93 per pound for a product that is 50 percent sugar?

The fact that these cereals are fortified does not redeem them. A sugar-coated vitamin is still not an economical choice. Stick with the simple cereals. All the hot cereals are good buys and especially welcome in winter. Rolled oats are an excellent choice. Recent studies have suggested that oat bran may have benefits in reducing the risk of certain types of colon cancers. It is a low-cost, easy-to-prepare, and delicious breakfast cereal.

Generally, cereals to be cooked are cheaper than ready-to-eat cereals and they are often more nutritious. It is less expensive to add your own raisins and other dried fruits than to have the manufacturer do it for you. Ready-to-eat cereals without sugar are cheaper than those with sugar and are a better nutritional buy. Cereal in individual packages are more than three times more expensive than the same cereal in large boxes.

Tortillas

Tortillas are the bread of Mexico. Mexican food is the most popular ethnic food in America today. Tortillas are high in fiber and contain trace amounts of calcium. In many states they are enriched, and are sold by the dozen.

I lived in the Mission District in San Francisco for many years and was lucky enough to get fresh tortillas. In Mexico I went to the market each morning to buy them while they were still hot. I bought a dozen and a half. The half was to eat on the walk home! Jennifer's favorite main dish is beans and tortillas.

Rice

Rice is economical and versatile. It is easy to prepare and its bland flavor combines well with many ingredients. It can be long-, medium-, or short-grain.

Regular white rice has been milled to remove the hull, germ, and practically all the bran. This removes some of the vitamins and minerals. Therefore, buy only enriched white rice.

Parboiled rice is even better. It is treated by a special steam-pressure process before milling. This forces the vitamins and minerals from the hull, bran, and germ into the starchy part of the grain, so that much of the natural vitamin and mineral content is retained after milling. It is then also enriched. Parboiled rice does take a little longer to cook than regular rice and is a bit chewier.

Precooked or minute rice has been cooked and dried. It takes less preparation time than regular white rice but costs more.

Brown rice is whole grain rice from which only the hull and a small amount of the bran has been removed. It retains more of the natural vitamins and minerals than white rice. It has a delicious nutlike flavor and a slightly chewy texture. If your family has not tasted brown rice, try it out on them. If they still prefer white rice as a side dish, use brown rice in your casseroles and soups.

Potatoes

Like turkeys, corn, and cranberries, potatoes are a native American food. There are over fifty varieties, twelve of which we commonly find in grocery stores. They have various names but are usually also labeled by use. New potatoes are best when boiled. Baking potatoes are just that. And general purpose potatoes can serve all purposes.

Potatoes are 99 percent fat free and remain so when baked or boiled. Their reputation as a "fattening" food comes from the company they keep rather than from any attribute of their own. When they are smothered in butter, dressed in sour cream, or covered in gravy, calories are added by association.

Eating a plain potato is no more fattening than eating a pear. Turning it into French fries or tater tots or fried spudettes can quadruple the calories. It can also double the cost if you buy these items in the frozen food section.

Mashed or creamed potatoes can be a nice change of pace from plain baked or boiled. However, the cream and butter add calories. Instead use skim or low-fat milk (or evaporated skim or whole milk) to keep fat and calories to a minimum. (I leave the peels on and whip them in too. This adds flavor and saves time.)

A baked potato topped with grated cheese and served with a salad can make a whole meal. Many fast-food operations are capitalizing on this menu idea. Beware of the toppings they offer. Again, many are fat-filled and fattening.

Potatoes store well so you can buy them in bulk usually at considerable savings per pound. Do not wash them before storing. Store them in a dark, dry, cool place—not the refrigerator. They will keep for several months.

Cakes and Cookies

In the thirties and forties, cakes and cookies were a staple part of our diet. We engaged in more physical types of work than we do today and could use the extra calories. Curiously, recipes in that era also contained less sugar and fat than today's recipes.

Increasingly today, cakes and cookies are purchased rather than prepared at home. The freezer department provides ready-to-thaw-and-serve cakes with icings. In-store bakeries offer plain and decorated cakes. It costs more than twice as much to purchase a cake as to make it at home from scratch.

There is little value in spending your money to purchase or your time to make sweets. Most of us do not need the empty calories. We most certainly do not need sweets to poke mindlessly into our mouths as we watch our favorite situation comedies.

As has been said before, if you are going to indulge your wallet and your waistline, buy a really fine dessert, serve it like a king's meal, and thoroughly pay attention to it as you consume it.

PROTEIN FOOD GROUPS

As was mentioned when we discussed the role of protein in health, Americans eat more protein, particularly from animal sources, than they need. Protein foods are costly. By cutting back on protein intake, we can save dollars. Because animal sources of protein come naturally packaged with fat, especially saturated fats and cholesterol, we can save calories and avoid fats when we eat fewer and leaner cuts of meat.

Beef

There are two criteria for buying beef: the quality grade and the cut. Tenderness is determined by the amount of fat and fat marbling in the meat. The grade reflects the amount of fat. The cut reflects the location from which the meat is taken. The less exercised the tissue from which the cut is made, the fatter it will be. The more fat in a cut, the more juicy, tender, and flavorful it is.

There are three quality grades. *Prime* is the most expensive and is most often sold to restaurants. It is the highest in fat content. These are the standing rib roasts which you see in menu photos with a thick layer of fat on the outside and plenty of fat marbling inside.

Choice grade is sold most often in our supermarkets. *Good* grade meats are low in fat, lean cuts. They are often used by manufacturers for soups and stews. It is not as easy to find good grade meat for purchase.

A prime grade steak has more calories than a choice or good grade steak because it has more fat. It also costs more. Good grade is the least expensive and has the least fat. The most tender cuts are rib roasts, steaks, loin cuts like porterhouse, T-bone, club, and sirloin. They are the most expensive cuts. Next are moderately tender cuts, rump roasts, sirloin tip roasts, blade chuck roasts and steaks, top round roasts and steaks, and shoulder cut roasts. These are moderately expensive. The least expensive cuts are shoulder arm chuck roasts and steaks, flank steaks, bottom round and eye-of-the-round steaks and roasts and brisket. These last cuts must be cooked by moist heat methods.

If your family eats red meats, it makes economic and nutritional good sense to limit use to once weekly and to favor the leaner cut. It can also save time. A beef stew can be put in your slow cooker to simmer all day while you are at work or doing other activities. Adding vegetables to the stew will extend the meat to yield more servings. Leftovers can be frozen for future meals.

Pork

Until ten years or so ago, pork was thought to be a fatty meat and few people ate it. Today, due to changes in breeding and feeding, pork is a much leaner meat and is still tender. Prices are often less than those of beef. It is graded like beef, with prime grade being the fattiest.

We were also cautious about eating fresh pork because we feared trichina, a worm which can grow in contaminated pork.

We tended to eat pork most often as hams and breakfast meats which have been cured or smoked to kill the trichina.

Cured hams have been preserved by mechanically pumping a solution of salt, sugar, and sodium nitrate through them. Smoked hams are smoked to an internal temperature of 140 degrees F to kill trichina. They must still be cooked at home. Fully cooked or ready-to-eat hams need no further cooking. Canned hams may be cured and/or smoked and are ready-to-eat.

Trichinosis is rarely a problem today due to the more sanitary conditions under which pork is raised and butchered. However, I must say that I remain skeptical about the safety of nitrites which are used not only in hams but in bacon, sausage, corned beef, pastrami, hot dogs, and several other cured meats. Nitrites are added to protect us from contamination of the meat, yet there is evidence that nitrites are carcinogenic.

If you like these meats, keep their use to a limit in your diet. Or substitute the breakfast meats and hot dogs, and so forth, which are made without nitrites. Remember that they are still high in fat and sodium. All things in excess are potentially harmful. All things in moderation limit their potential harm. Do keep these meats to a moderate amount and frequency if you eat them.

Lamb

Lamb is often a good buy and can give flavorful variety to your meals. My Utah cousins are Mormons for whom lamb and mutton (older, tougher meat) are standard fare. My aunt uses it to replace beef in recipes for everything from potpies to chili. Friends in Fresno, California, who are Armenian, likewise use lamb rather than beef as their primary animal protein. Shish kabobs are popular street-vended snacks in New York City.

Because most lamb is from animals that are less than one year old, it is usually tender. It is graded like beef with prime, choice, and good grades. The most expensive cuts are lamb chops, leg of lamb, and rack of lamb.

Poultry

Poultry is graded differently from red meats. All poultry—chicken, turkey, duck, goose, and guinea—are either Grade A or Grade B. Grade A is a fully fleshed and meaty bird with a well-finished fat layer and no blemishes or marks. A Grade B bird is less well finished and blemish-free and slightly less meaty.

Tenderness is determined by age. Young birds are more tender than older ones. (My father disagrees. He thinks that "old birds" are far more gentle, tender, and less demanding of their men. But that's a bird of a different color!)

Young chickens may be labeled young chicken, Rock Cornish game hen, broiler, fryer, roaster, or capon. Young turkeys may be labeled young turkey, young hen, young tom, or fryer-roaster. Young ducks may be labeled duckling, young duckling, broiler duckling, fryer duckling, or roaster duckling. These can all be barbecued, roasted, or broiled. (Remember, no frying!)

Mature, less tender birds may be labeled mature, old, hen, stewing, or fowl chicken. Older turkeys may be labeled mature, yearling, or old. Mature ducks, geese, and guineas may be labeled mature or old.

Generally, poultry is a versatile and good buy. The meat itself is not fatty, although the skin is. In fact, the majority of fat and cholesterol present in poultry is found in the skin. Removing the skin before cooking will reduce fat and cholesterol content.

It would seem that chicken or turkey parts are better buys than the whole bird. After all, you avoid wings, tail, neck, and other parts which are not family favorites. In fact you may pay up to 40–50 percent more for someone else to cut the chicken into parts for you. The parts which are in less demand can be used to make chicken salad, chicken soup, stew, or potpies.

Prepared Meats

When purchasing prepared products with meat in them, read the label to determine how much meat you are actually buying. There is no need to pay meat prices for a product that contains less meat than its name might suggest. For example, "gravy with beef" contains more gravy than beef. "Beef with gravy" contains more beef and is a better buy.

It is surprising to learn what the actual meat content of many familiar products are. It is not required that the percentage of meat in the product be stated on the label. The government does set minimum standards for the amount of meat which must be in the product. It is often low. As an example, in table 6.11 are listed popular products with the percentage of meat contained.

TABLE 6.11 PERCENT MEAT IN VARIOUS PRODUCTS

Food Name	% Meat or Poultry
Beans with bacon or ham in sauce	12% bacon or ham
Beef almondine with vegetables	18% beef
Beef with gravy	50% beef
Breakfast sausage	About 43½% meat; no more than 50% fat; may also contain up to 3½% binders and 3% water
Burrito	15% meat
Chili con carne	40% meat
Chili con carne with beans	25% meat
Chili Mac	16% meat
Chow mein vegetables with meat	12% meat
Chow mein vegetables with meat and noodles	8% meat
Dinner—frozen meal containing meat	25% meat
Egg roll with meat	10% meat
Enchilada with meat	15% meat
Entrée: meat or meat product plus one vegetable	50% meat
Gravy and Swiss steak	35% meat
Gravy and Yankee pot roast	35% meat
Ham and cheese spread	25% ham
Ham salad	35% ham
Knish	15% meat
Kreplach	20% meat
Lasagne with meat sauce	6% meat
Lima beans with ham or bacon in sauce	12% ham or bacon
Macaroni and beef in sauce	12% beef
Meat loaf (baked or oven-ready)	65% meat and no more than 12% cereal products
Meat pie	25% beef
Meat ravioli	10% meat
Meat soups	
Ready to eat	5% meat
Condensed	10% meat
Noodles or dumplings with poultry	6% poultry
Pizza with sausage	12% sausage
Poultry à la king	20% poultry
Poultry almondine	50% poultry
Poultry Brunswick stew	12% poultry
Poultry chop suey	4% poultry
Poultry dinner—frozen	18% poultry
Poultry pie	14% poultry
Poultry salad	25% poultry

TABLE 6.11 (*cont.*)

Food Name	% Meat or Poultry
Shepherd's pie	25% meat
Sloppy joe	35% meat
Spaghetti with meat or meatballs in sauce	12% meat
Tamale	25% meat

Source: USDA, *Meat and Poultry Products—A Consumer Guide to Content and Labeling Requirements*, July 1981.

Fish

Brain food fish may or may not be, but high in good-quality protein, low in both fat and calories it is. Even those fish which are high in fat—salmon, herring, mackerel, bluefish, and butterfish—are lower in fat and calories than most beef and pork.

At one time fish was considerably lower in price per pound than red meats or poultry. Today many fish are still excellent buys but the price differential has narrowed. You will find fresh fish, thawed frozen fish, frozen fish, and frozen-prepared fish. Fresh is best in texture and flavor when cooked. Frozen which you thaw at home or fish which was frozen then thawed by the grocer have a slightly grainy texture when cooked.

Frozen breaded fish or fish frozen with a sauce adds cost and calories. By law, up to 35 percent of a breaded product can be breading and other ingredients. You may pay fish prices for bread. To get your dollars' worth, buy plain frozen fish and bread it yourself. You will get more fish, less bread, and save money and calories.

Fish deteriorates far more quickly than red meats or poultry. It must be handled with care and kept under refrigeration. Fresh fish should be used within two days of purchase. If you do not plan to use the fish immediately, it is better to buy the fish already frozen than to freeze it yourself.

Fish requires very little cooking. Many people overcook it, then complain that fish is dry, papery, and tasteless. It is only when it is overcooked. Follow recipe timing instructions closely. If the recipe says broil for 10 minutes do not broil for 20.

Eggs

There are three consumer grades for eggs based on interior quality of the egg and appearance of the egg shell. U.S. Grade AA eggs have thick whites, firm and perfect yolks, and clean, unbroken shells.

The grade most common in grocery stores is U.S. Grade A. They have reasonably firm whites, yolks that are high (not flat) and practically free from defects, and clean, unbroken shells.

Grade B eggs are seldom found in retail stores. They are used by food manufacturers in cooking and baking. They have thinner whites, flat yolks, and broken or stained shells.

Most grocers have eggs in four sizes. Since a unit is one egg and the eggs are different sizes, it is difficult to compare unit price. To see which is the best buy, use the chart below. If large eggs are selling for $1.20 per dozen and small for 90 cents per dozen, which is the best buy? From table 6.12 you see that they actually cost the same, 80 cents per pound.

TABLE 6.12 EGG PRICES CALCULATED BY POUND

Price per lb (16 oz)	Price per Dozen Small (18 oz)	Medium (21 oz)	Large (24 oz)	X-large (27 oz)
.60	.675	.79	.90	1.01
.63	.71	.83	.95	1.07
.665	.75	.875	1.00	1.125
.70	.79	.92	1.05	1.18
.73	.825	.96	1.10	1.24
.765	.86	1.005	1.15	1.29
.80	.90	1.05	1.20	1.35
.83	.94	1.09	1.25	1.405

If table 6.12 is too complex, an easier method is to subtract ⅛ of the price from the larger size and compare this price to the price of the next size. Buy whichever is cheapest. For example, if large eggs are $1.40 per dozen, medium would have to cost less than $1.22 to be a better buy. ($1.40 − (⅛ of 1.40) = $1.22)

Egg Substitutes

Egg substitutes, marketed under various names, are eggs without the yolk. That is, they are egg whites to which fat and food coloring have been added to make them look like whole, beaten eggs. They are sold for people who must severely restrict their intake of cholesterol.

Unless your doctor has told you to control cholesterol intake strictly and you feel that you cannot live without eggs, it is probably not necessary to use egg substitutes. Eggs do have approximately 250 milligrams of cholesterol per yolk, a high amount. However, two or three per week (NOTE: I did not say per day!) will not unduly increase your blood cholesterol levels.

Beans, The Musical Food

Ten years ago beans were common in our homes as beanbag chairs to slump in, dangle over, and curl around while we watched TV. Some inventive seamstresses made comical beanbag dolls (usually frogs with mouths that you could stick your finger into) for Christmas presents.

But no one *ate* beans. Beans had a very bad reputation. They were for poor folks, down, out, struggling across state borders, *Grapes of Wrath*—fashion in search of a job. They were for soldiers out on military maneuvers, in harsh conditions, protecting liberty. But they weren't for polite folk. After all, they cause gas.

To date, none of our agricultural botanists has bred a gas-free bean. The gas is caused by the failure of our digestive system to break down one of the complex carbohydrates contained in beans. When that carbohydrate reaches the large intestine, bacteria that normally live there break it down, releasing gas.

There does not seem to be any way to avoid the gas. Adding baking soda to the boiling water is rumored to work. I am not convinced that it does, so I do not bother to add it.

If flatulence (the medical term for gas) is a major concern for you, select beans from the high end of the following list, number one as most gaseous and ten as least.

1. Soybeans
2. Pink beans
3. Black beans
4. Pinto Beans
5. California small white beans
6. Great northern beans
7. Lima beans, baby
8. Garbanzo beans
9. Lima beans, large
10. Black-eyed peas

Dried beans, peas, and legumes are the least expensive source of protein available in the world today. They have the added nutritional benefit of being virtually fat free.

Beans are not complete proteins. That is, they do not contain all of the essential amino acids. This is simply solved by mixing beans with other vegetables which contain the essential amino acids which they are missing or by including a bit of meat, cheese, egg, or other animal protein with them.

There are dozens of varieties: black, red, pink, and white, kidney, soy, mung, lima, navy, pea, pinto, cranberry, black-eye, garbanzo, and others. All are relatively bland in flavor and will absorb the flavor of other ingredients, including spices and herbs, with which they are cooked. It is for this reason that they are among the most versatile of cooking ingredients.

I keep a pot of cooked beans available in the refrigerator just as some of you keep meat in the freezer. Beans are substituted for meat in many of my recipes, and in others, beans become the central ingredients.

My lasagna contains either kidney or pinto beans instead of meat. Minestrone has no meat but extra red beans or garbanzos. Enchilada pie, tacos, burritos, and tostados are all meatless and bean-filled. A mixture of beans makes a delicious "meat" loaf. Leftovers can be sliced to fill sandwiches. Seasoned with cumin, turmeric, and coriander, beans take on the flavor of the Middle East. With cumin, chili, and cilantro they go south of the border. With garlic, olive oil, oregano, and basil they become Sicilian sensations. And with curry and chutney they bring us the essence of India.

If your taste buds tire of all these gastronomical variations, you can always have simple "Okie" beans. My father is chef par excellence of "Okie" beans. He puts beans and water on to cook in his slow cooker. After several hours he adds a block of frozen chili and cooks them another hour or so. A pan of homemade corn bread and a tossed salad complete the meal.

I usually visit California at least once every three months. A particularly long five months had elapsed at one point. I arrived home just before midnight and found a pot of Daddy's beans and a pan of corn bread. They were so delicious that I ate four bowls (really! four cupfuls!). Even someone without a gas problem with beans produces gas after four bowls of beans, and by 4:00 A.M. my poor stomach was in pain!

Peanut Butter

Peanut butter is the source and wellspring of all intelligent life in the universe. Or at least, so I have always believed! It is also a very American food. It was developed here by the brilliant scientist, George Washington Carver, and has not become a popular food outside the United States.

If you are already a peanut butter fan, the world for you is divided into "smoothies" and "crunchy" or "nutty grinds." And you know that the two personality types are incompatible. A "smoothie" would NEVER date a "nutty" and vice versa. The consequences are too grave! What if they were to fall in love? Can two-texture families survive? Or is the inconvenience of living a dual-purchasing-pattern life, and the risk of having to consume the other's texture when your own supply is depleted, just too drastic to consider? Should one of you convert? How should you raise the children?

If you are a fan you will probably prefer products made with 100 percent peanuts, called old-fashioned or natural. These are made with just peanuts and perhaps a bit of salt. They are very peanutty in flavor. The peanut oil usually separates and rises to the top of the jar which makes the last spoonful of peanut butter a little dry and hard to spread.

Most peanut butters contain 90 percent peanuts, the minimum limit set by law. The remaining 10 percent can be sweeteners, hardened vegetable oil, and salt. When hydrogenated vegetable oil is added, the product is homogenized to keep the oil from separating from the peanuts and to make it spread easier.

Peanut butter is a great snack food as well as a great sandwich filler. It can be smoothed onto celery sticks, apple quarters, or banana slices, stuffed into dried dates, or eaten straight out of the jar with a spoon.

PROCESSED, PACKAGED, FLUFFED, AND PUFFED

You can spot a fake fur or a copy of a famous painting without much difficulty. If you are in doubt, you can check the price. Minks and Mona Lisas do not sell for bargain-basement prices plus tax.

Fake foods are not always as easy to spot. They are often made to look like and are packaged just like the real thing. They are sold right alongside the authentics and they may cost about the same.

You may not even be aware of foods that you already use which are fabricated versions of real foods. Coffee creamers look like cream after you stir the powders into your coffee but they never saw a cow. They are nondairy made from polyunsaturated soy oil and sugar. Whipped dessert toppings have similar ingredients.

Hot dogs made from turkey and turkey rolls made from soy protein sit next to the real thing in the meat case. Candy without sugar, fruit drinks without fruit, bacon bits that never saw a pork belly, and high-fiber bread made with wood shavings, all invite our purchase.

Alternatively, traditional foods may be offered to us in new fangle-dangle forms. You can buy anchovy paste, mustard, and fish pâtés in tubes that look like toothpaste. You can buy perfectly uniform "potato" chips in a can. They are not deep-fat, fried potato slices at all but potato paste.

Until World War II, scientists concerned themselves largely with finding better techniques to preserve food—canning, refrigeration, cellophane wrapping. Today they are more concerned with producing new foods in new forms with new and unusual containers. Their efforts have moved food production from the farm to the factory.

What is the cost of these innovations? More than half of our food dollars go to purchase processed and packaged foods. We spend over $12 billion annually on fabricated foods alone.

Some of this processing provides us with built-in labor and time-savings. Some of it merely adds ingredients which are best eaten in small amounts or not at all. Some of the items rob us of our cash and leave us with little positive health benefits and possibly some health risks.

Convenience Foods

In my grandmother's youth, women planted, harvested, and preserved most of the family food supply. Grandma had a cellar for potatoes, carrots, and other root vegetables; a pantry for her canned fruits, vegetables, and preserves; an ice box for home-butchered meats and homemade sausages; and cows and chickens to supply fresh milk, cheese, cream, and eggs.

Among her first concessions to modernization was the use of

canned vegetables. Grandpa sold the cows when the last of the children left home. And today Grandma even buys an occasional frozen dinner.

Her life was obviously not like yours and mine. Over 42 percent of us work outside our homes either part or full time. As a consequence, 95 percent of Americans purchase the majority of their food supply. The farm-fresh foods that Grandma produced are now processed by large factories. If we make preserves or can vegetables it is more likely to be hobby than necessity.

In addition to preserving basic food items for us, the food industry also provides us with foods which are in part or in whole ready to heat and eat. Sales of convenience foods have grown steadily and now account for fully half of the typical grocery store's sales.

"Convenience" foods, those that have been premixed or partially or fully preprepared, may save time and effort. Someone else has done the work for you. The question is, how much time have they really saved you and can you afford their help?

Some convenience foods are such a part of our lives that we may forget the labor which is built into them. Many of these are penny-wise purchases. They may be less costly because they use canned or frozen ingredients which cut down costs due to spoilage. Some are less costly because the manufacturer can buy in bulk and pass savings on to us.

Convenience foods that you can count on to save you time and money include:

Instant mashed potatoes	Preshredded packaged coconut
Canned cranberry sauce	Frozen or canned orange juice
Bottled lemon or lime juice	Frozen and canned shrimp
Cake mixes	Instant milk
Pancake and waffle mixes	Canned pineapple in own juice

When the food items become more complicated, the cost-convenience trade-off begins to be questionable. Some do not really save all that much time. Many are not nutritionally equivalent to their made-from-scratch counterparts. For example, frozen TV dinners can vary from 15 percent to 100 percent higher in cost than the same meal made at home.

Convenience foods are great when an unexpected guest stays for dinner, when you arrive home exhausted and the cupboard is otherwise bare, or for family meals when you are away. But as a steady diet they can be hard on the budget and in some cases provide less nutrition than homemade foods. I make my own frozen dinners and entrées. You'll see why.

Convenience foods are not a good buy if they are short on nutrients. A serving of canned chicken chow mein contains 3½ ounces of chicken. Chicken chow mein made at home from a conventional recipe contains 6 ounces of chicken. Canned beef stew might contain 4 ounces of beef while a homemade version has twice as much.

Some frozen dinners have meat substitutes added to the product. These substitutes, made from textured vegetable protein (called TVP) are safe and healthy but contain less protein than the meat for which they substitute. They are also a less expensive ingredient than meat. If you are paying meat prices for a meat-loaf TV dinner, you should get meat.

Further, many convenience foods have levels of salt, sugar, and fats added which far exceed that of a traditional recipe. Some TV dinners have as much as 1600 milligrams of sodium, an excessive amount for a single meal. Many of the dinners have sauces over the meats adding unnecessarily to your fat and calorie intake.

A USDA price comparison study revealed that in two out of three instances, the cost of convenience foods was at least 15 cents per serving more than the cost of homemade. Among beef products, a beef pie costs 20 cents more than making it at home, a beef dinner 27 cents more, a meat-loaf dinner 54 cents more, and a serving of lasagne 35 cents more.

Remember, these are per serving cost differences. Chicken a la king cost 20 cents more per serving, a fried chicken dinner 41 cents more, and a turkey dinner 52 cents more. The total increased cost for a family meal for four could range from less than $1 more to over $2 more.

You may feel that the added cost is worth the time saved. The question then becomes, is time actually saved? I asked a high-school home economics class in Pittsburgh to do a price, time, and taste comparison for me for three convenience foods: tuna noodle casserole, pancakes, and chicken cacciatore. Each was compared in canned, frozen, dry-packaged, and scratch form.

We filmed their findings for one of my television segments on *PM/Evening Magazine*. The students were most impressed by how much more flavor the scratch products had. Even in blind tests, they preferred the scratch products for color, texture, and taste.

Next they were impressed with the comparative prices.

Scratch cost less in all cases. What most surprised them, however, was the time element. Scratch method took only 4–6 minutes longer to prepare the tuna and chicken dishes and 2–3 minutes longer to prepare pancakes from start to on the plate than frozen or canned. The difference between scratch and dry-packaged was even less. The students unanimously felt that the superior quality and cost savings of the scratch products were worth the few extra minutes of preparation.

To boil rice in a pouch requires that you get out a pan, fill it with water, open the box, and drop in the bag. To make rice from scratch requires that you get out the pan, measure water and rice, and add them to the water. To make a plain omelet from a carton requires the same skill as to make one from fresh eggs. Even Jennifer at eight can crack eggs into a skillet.

If it takes 10 or even 20 minutes longer to prepare a meal from scratch, is it worth it? Your time is definitely money, but you may save less time than you think. Further, you might be trading off taste, texture, and color appeal and possibly nutritional quality to save a few minutes.

If you are protesting that one of the reasons you use convenience foods is you do not know how to make chicken Kiev, consider this. Home preparation of many so-called convenience foods takes no more skill than it takes to pop the pouch in the pan.

Advertisements encourage fears and feelings of inadequacy by suggesting that we cannot cook rice without clumps or fry chicken as well as some fictional character pictured on the package. You might be surprised if you looked up the recipe for some of your favorite convenience foods. Many of them are not as difficult to prepare as their foreign names are to pronounce!

Convenience foods do have a place in our fast-paced lives. Even Henry Ford figured out the advantages of having someone other than his employees make his car floorboards and sides. But he did not make the decision blindly.

Be conscious of what you are purchasing. Are you buying someone else's labor? Could any of that labor be delegated to a family member? Are you buying someone else's cooking skill? Is the implied skill real or imaginery (as in cracking eggs!)? Are you buying time? If so, how much real time are you buying and at what cost? What are you sacrificing in addition to your pocketbook in the exchange?

No manager of a major company would make a purchase decision without going through an analysis similar to the above. Often the differences which they are analyzing in cost per item are fractions of a cent, not even dollars!

Fifteen cents per serving may not look like a great deal of money. Added up over a year it could provide the family with a nice little vacation or you with a new winter coat!

Fabricated Foods

Fabricated foods substitute for and resemble traditional foods in taste, texture, appearance, and usage. They are sometimes lower in fat, calories, and cholesterol than the counterparts they replace. But more often they are higher in sodium and sugar, full of preservatives and artificial flavors and colors, and lower in essential nutrients than the natural food which they imitate or replace. Their appeal is that they can be cheaper than the real thing and they last longer on the shelf.

For some people who need to severely restrict their intake of dietary fats or sugar, these imitation foods may offer a way to enjoy old favorite foods periodically. Someone on a very strict fat-controlled diet for heart disease might enjoy whipped topping on his or her fresh strawberries. However, there are risks, even for people whose health might benefit.

Imitation foods do not really duplicate nature. These foods may look and taste "real" but they fall short on several counts. First, we have not yet identified all of the important constituents of natural foods and therefore we cannot imitate them with 100 percent accuracy.

Second, manufacturers commonly add only 8 to 12 of the more than 45 nutrients which we know to be essential to human health. A diet with a high concentration of fabricated foods risks low or inadequate intakes of essential nutrients. You cannot compensate by taking a vitamin supplement. The supplements also contain only a dozen or so nutrients.

Salt and sugar are often added to fabricated foods in high quantities. Salt may be added for flavor or it may be a residual of the manufacturing process. For example, textured vegetable protein used to make mock chicken and breakfast sausage imitations (usually called "links") contains up to six times more salt than its natural counterpart.

Color and flavor additives and preservatives complete the cornucopia of contents in these manufactured foods. They are sometimes used in processed natural foods, too, but not at the levels found in processed foods. For example, coloring makes butter brighter, oranges oranger, and cherries redder.

Unfortunately, reading the name on the label may not tell you if the product is fake. The Food and Drug Administration, which regulates food labeling, does not have consistent rules for fabricated foods. For example, salad dressing does not have to be called "imitation mayonnaise" because a standard of identity was established by the FDA to specify what ingredients salad dressing can contain.

The FDA rules on this matter allow leeway in stretching the truth. Imitation crumbled bacon can be labeled "baco-bits"—a name which is highly suggestive of the real product but avoids the word "imitation."

Some product names suggest a natural ingredient when none exists. Boo Berries, a children's breakfast cereal, suggests that blueberries might be in the box. You will find artificially flavored blue marshmallows, but no berries.

Other products do not offer themselves as imitations of real foods though they may suggest that a real ingredient is contained in the product. Many snack foods fall into this category. Break-fast toaster squares look as if they are filled with fruit preserves. They are not. The filling is a sugary paste of artificial fruit complete with the flavor, aroma, and texture of real fruit.

Among the marvels of modern manufacturing are snack cakes. The Twinkie, the first of these man-made marvels, has been all but eclipsed in popularity by a cache of concoctions in flavors from apple to strawberry. Their ingredients read like a postgraduate chemistry textbook.

It is amazing that the products even look like cake or hold together. I certainly cannot imagine how to bake such tiny cakes with so much sugary-gooey stuffing. I am further amazed that anyone would eat them. A dear friend of mine swears that Moonpies, which he calls the mascot food of Nashville, are delicious. In deference to him I tasted them. They were like sticky cardboard.

These fabricated fun foods are high in sugar and fat and low in overall vitamin, mineral, protein, and fiber content. They have been called empty calorie foods because they provide calories and little else. For many of these novelty foods, sugar contributes as high as one-half of the calories contained.

If you crave sweets, a piece of fruit is a better nutritional buy (see page 169). If you must have sugar, it is far less expensive to buy it by the bagful and sprinkle a bit over your peaches or bake a few homemade oatmeal cookies than it is to buy these cute-named, cleverly advertised enticements.

As a rule of thumb, I would avoid fabricated foods or keep their use to a minimum. They are costly and provide little return on your investment.

NUTRITIONALLY ECONOMIC FOODS— THE VERY BEST BUYS

There was a game we played as children in which you had to name an item you would take with you on a picnic. You said, "I'm going on a picnic and I'm taking a radish." The leader, who knew the secret, would then tell you whether or not you could go. The game proceeded around the circle repeatedly until everyone guessed what the secret was to selecting an item so that he or she could go on the picnic. (My editor insisted that I tell you the answer! The item taken has to begin with the same letter as the first letter in your name. Alice can take apples but not bananas.)

In a serious study which captured my imagination rather like that game, Dr. George Briggs, at the University of California, Department of Nutritional Sciences, asked the question, given that food dollars are dwindling, what foods are the most economical buys. Had you asked a dozen shoppers that question, they might well have come up with guesses as lame as game players trying to figure out why they can't go on the picnic.

Forty food items in the San Francisco area in March 1982 were priced. Using a computer, the researchers calculated the amount that $1 could purchase, the amount of energy, and the contribution per dollar's worth of food for the following nutrients: protein, calcium, phosphorus, magnesium, zinc, copper, iron, total vitamin A activity, thiamine, riboflavin, niacin, vitamin B-6, pantothenic acid, free folacin, vitamin B-12, and vitamin C.

They then did a nutrient-cost ratio to determine which foods were the most nutritionally economic buys. Here's what they found (table 6.13).

TABLE 6.13 MOST NUTRIENT/DENSE FOODS
PER DOLLAR SPENT

Spinach	Tofu
Beef liver	Dry roasted peanuts
Fresh tomatoes	Eggs
Canned tuna (in water)	Fresh carrots
Nonfat and low-fat milk	

So, the answer to the question, "I'm going to the supermarket, what should I buy?" involves no tricks. These are basic staples which yield good buys for the buck.

7. Management Maneuvers —Saving Time and Money

The two scarcest commodities in our culture are time and money. We complain of having time but no money to spend, or money but no time to spend it, or, more frequently in today's double-digit inflation era, neither time nor money!

Both can be magically expanded beyond economist Milton Friedman's theory of elasticity through planning and delegation. Just as your fingers can do the walking through the Yellow Pages to save you time and effort, so can the "power of the pen" save you money and time. The first, last, and most critical maneuver to gaining control is to put TIME where it counts: in *planning*.

TIME IS MONEY

Most of us believe that there will never be enough time in a day, even in a 25-hour day, to do all the things we want and need to do in the way we want to do them. The truth may be, however, that there is more than enough time.

Time is relative. There is no such thing as "time" in and of itself. There is only the relationship between time, energy, and purpose. The test of time is how much is expended, with what energy, toward what end.

We talk about time in quantitative terms: "There goes another wasted morning!" "If only I had started this project earlier!" "I am out of time and late again!" The quantity seems always to be less than is needed. This too is a matter of perception.

When we are having fun, we pay little attention to time, and before we know it, our ball gown and glass slippers are about to disappear. When we are stuck in the middle of drudgery, time drags.

According to Mr. Webster, time does not have the ability to fly or drag. It is merely "a nonspatial continuum in which events occur in apparently irreversible succession from the past through the present to the future."

Our use of time often has those characteristics too . . . nonspatial, irreversible, and likely to be used in the future in the same way it was in the past! To get control of time, we need to begin to think in terms of how well, toward what end, and with what result or reward we want to use our time.

We need a plan. The plan needs to be more than a list of activities for the day. It needs to rank activities in order of their importance, their difficulty or ease to accomplish, the purpose of the activity, AND the person to whom the activity should be delegated.

We need to know:

1. Things that MUST be done and why
2. Things that we WANT to get done by a certain time and why
3. Things that would be NICE to do, if and when there is time
4. How and by whom to get them done

We can now begin to match time with responsibility. How much time will it take for each item on the MUST list? Is there a more energy-efficient way to accomplish it? Can it be delegated to someone else in the family? Can it be delegated to someone outside the family and if so, at what cost?

Unfortunately, according to time management experts, we spend most of our time doing those things which produce the least results. The Pareto Time Principle states that 80 percent of our time is devoted to 20 percent of the results we want in our lives. In the remaining 20 percent, we attempt to accomplish those 80 percent of things which must be done.

Certainly routine tasks take time. However, the amount of time they actually require may be considerably less than is spent. Below when we discuss shopping and kitchen cleanup timesavers, we will see two areas where "time-allocated" can become "time-alligator," swallowing hours.

Time robbers lurk in our lives waiting to steal minutes from us. Lack of meal plans for the week may lead to repeated trips to the grocer to pick up items to complete a meal. An unorganized shopping list, or no list at all, means minutes lost in the market, wandering aimlessly about, returning to aisles you have already been down to get items that you forgot when you first passed them on the shelf.

Making a trip out of your way to pick up needed food items that are on your husband's route home is a waste of your time. Setting the dinner table yourself when your five-year-old could do it robs you of time and delays dinner while everyone waits for Mom to do it.

Distractions often delay us. When our attention is divided we are less efficient. If we are watching television while we work, we may not notice the rice boiling over on the stove. Cleaning up creates work. Phone calls from friends and demands from children can sidetrack us.

We have a telephone answering machine which we use to screen calls. If friends call while I am rushing to complete a job, I do not pick up the phone. I let the machine take their message and I return their call when I have time to relax and enjoy being with them.

Using inefficient work methods wastes time and money. Squeezing oranges for breakfast juice is not efficient or economical. Hand slicing five different vegetables for a simple supper soup instead of using a food processor robs you of time. Having kitchen appliances which you rarely or never use robs you of money, time, and kitchen space.

The key to controlling time and money is planning. The skeleton of a family food and nutrition plan is meal menus. From that we build shopping lists, inventories of nonperishable staples and perishable goods, preparation schedules, and delegation lists.

CUTTING SHOPPING TIME

Interviews of 4000 shoppers in 200 supermarkets done by Point of Purchase Advertising Institute showed that the average American shopper spends about 32 minutes in the supermarket. If you make more than one trip weekly, the minutes multiply.

Several rules of thumb can increase your speed and efficiency when shopping.

Rule #1: Organize Your Shopping List

I find that the amount of time I spend in the supermarket is directly related to how well organized my shopping list is. If it is organized in the same order as the grocery store is laid out, then I spend less time retracing my steps to pick up items I overlooked on the list. If my list is random, so are my movements!

Rule #2: Shop Off-Hours

If at all possible, shop at off-hours. There will be less congestion in the aisles to slow you down and fewer people at the checkout point to wait behind.

Studies show that most shoppers like to visit the supermarket Thursday through Saturday during the midday. The least popular times to shop are evenings followed by Sunday through Wednesday during the day. When I worked in Washington, D.C., and had both a busy career and a crowded entertaining schedule, I frequently shopped at 7:00 A.M. when the market opened. This assured that all items which were needed for dinner were home and ready, even if I was delayed at work. It also avoided the long lines of people just after work who are buying their evening meal.

Rule #3: Buy Dry Goods Separate from Perishables

There are over 24,000 food items in the average grocery store today. Sorting through them can be a confusing and exhausting task. Many of these items are duplicates of others. For example, there may be canned peas under five different manufacturers' labels and in three different styles, for a total of fifteen selections.

Not all items offered are edible. In fact, many supermarkets today look more like department stores than grocery stores. To eliminate some of the choice confusion and several aisles in the store, twice yearly I purchase the majority of my dry goods. This saves repeated time spent in replenishing these items. Toilet paper, paper towels, bath soap, laundry soap, bleach, skin lotion, toothpaste, shaving cream, and a number of nonperishable goods like canned milk and canned tomato paste are purchased in bulk lots. And I tenaciously follow three golden rules:

Golden Rule #1

I never shop when I am hungry. Studies have shown that hungry shoppers not only purchase more than they had planned to, they also spend more time exploring aisles they do not normally frequent. It is probably the foraging instinct driving us in search of food.

Golden Rule #2

I do not take children or husband with me. Steven is an "Oh-isn't-this-interesting-why-don't-we-try-it?" shopper. If I do not keep a keen eye on the basket, it arrives at the checkout stand with a collection of curious condiments, newly arrived to this continent, expensive imported beer, and three varieties of salted snack chips at prices above the cost of meat.

Jennifer's eight-year-old eyes scan a different level of the shelves where marketing specialists in cahoots with the Sugar Plum Fairy have expertly placed sugar-laced, cartoon-character-laden boxes of candies disguised as cereals and snacks. She knows all of these characters and the attributes of their favorite food. She is ready to march them all home with us.

Unlike Steven, whose curiosity for the exotic and imported cannot be redirected, Jennifer can be distracted. When she does "help" me shop, I give her the task of fetching items within her reach. Now that she has become a whiz kid at mathematics, I also give her assignments to determine which of several items is the best buy. She likes this game and pays less attention to the pleas from her sugar-coated TV friends when she is engaged in choosing the best-priced apples.

Golden Rule #3

Finally, I do delegate shopping for special items when the store in which they are sold is closer to Steven's office than to mine. Or I wait to include these items in the menu when I know that I will be passing by that market. I never make a trip to an out-of-the-way store for only a single item. Too much time and transportation cost involved.

EQUIPMENT

You may be among those women who think that Hamilton Beach is a vacation resort and General Electric is a valuable stock to have in your portfolio. If so, you may need some advice on the basic equipment needed to produce balanced meals in minutes.

Alternatively, you may be a kitchen collector and the owner of every gadget, device, and appliance offered for sale or as a gift at Christmas over the past five years. If so, you may need to clear your counters of clutter and leave only the essentials.

Those of you in the first group will find stocking a kitchen a fairly easy task. Those of you in the second group will have far more difficulty. You are probably positive that someday you will in fact use that copper egg slicer, or make pots-du-crème in the fancy pottery you bought at a "French Kitchen" promotion at your local department store, or figure out how to get your melon baller to make perfect spheres rather than half-moons.

The first hurdle that collectors must overcome is the belief or hope that by "having" what great chefs have, their cooking will improve. Drawers and cupboards full of gadgets and gimmicks with attachments; books, magazines, and newsletters about them and the famous chefs who use them do not a gourmet cook make.

Kitchen supply and accessory stores are packed with such gadgetry. Many of the items are in themselves works of art. Others are truly useful if your menus frequently include items which require use of the gadget. A pastry blender is unnecessary if you use frozen pie crusts. If you never use fresh garlic, a garlic press is a novelty. For others these may be favorite and frequently used tools.

Unused and rarely used kitchen equipment robs our wallets as well as our wall and counter space. In a spurt of enthusiasm over winter soups, I once bought an elegant and expensive soup tureen. After the first week of excitement with my new toy, I retired it to the counter corner. Months later it went to the top of the cupboard and there it sat for three years collecting dust. It was a trophy to my compulsive misuse of capital! I finally gave it to a friend as a gift when the winter soup fever hit her. It is now sitting atop her cupboards.

When possible, choose items that have more than one use. Muffin pans can be used for many recipes, but corn-stick pans

cannot. A simple ring mold is more versatile than a fish-shaped mold. Cookware that can go from freezer to burner to table is a good investment.

For those of us on tight time schedules, what is needed are the basic tools which will turn the kitchen into an efficient production center with limited capital investment. By not tying our cash up in tools, we can devote more resources to the contents (ingredients) of the product.

Pots and Pans

My mother owned over five different sets of cookware in her lifetime. I have owned one set and see no reason to own more than that. Choose cookware carefully so that it will last. Avoid trendy wares that change color, design, pattern, and materials with the season. If you have not purchased pots and pans, look for the following:

Pots with water seal or snuggly fitted lids. This will allow for quick cooking at high temperatures to seal in freshness and flavor. Contents will steam-cook in a minimum amount of time to increase nutrient retention.

Cookware can be aluminum, steel—with or without copper bottom— copper, cast-iron, glass, porcelain, enamel-on-metal, or pottery. The cheapest is not the best buy. If it wears out soon, you have to replace it. If it burns and sticks or does not heat quickly, it is not a good buy. Good pots and pans last a long time and save food, fuel, and work for the cook.

Look for the gauge number on steel and aluminum cookware. The lower the gauge number, the thicker the metal. The bigger the number, the thinner the metal. Good cookware is 8, 10, or 12 gauge. Skillets should be heavier than the pots. The number will be on the purchase tag. If it is not attached, asked for it. Aluminum may stain from minerals in water and food. This does not mean that dangerous chemical reactions are taking place with your food.

Finishes and decorations, such as porcelain, acrylic enamel, and nonstick coating are often applied to cookware to reduce the reactions between the metal and foods. These finishes also make surfaces easier to clean, protect the base metal, and reduce food sticking.

Stainless steel is highly durable, easy to clean, and does not react with foods or detergents. However, it is a poor conductor of heat. Cookware made with stainless steel usually has a core of some other metal, often carbon, to increase heat conductivity.

Cast iron was the staple cookware of many a frontier home. It is still a favorite with many chefs. Cast iron is heavy to handle but is durable and relatively inexpensive. Its weight has its own usefulness. Mammy Yokum in Li'l Abner uses her cast-iron skillet to keep everyone under control.

Cast iron heats slowly and retains heat well. My family has a cast-iron 2-quart pot which we take on camping trips. After the pot and lid have been thoroughly heated in the campfire, you pop in homemade biscuits, put the hot lid on, and set it aside to "bake." Two of those biscuits and some of Grandma's jam and you are ready to climb the Sierras!

I swear by my dime-store cast-iron skillets. But they are not for everyone. If cast iron does not have a nonporous finishing coat, it takes particular care to prevent rust. It will also discolor eggs and foods containing acids, such as wine or vinegar, if the pot is not "seasoned." Seasoning is a process of oiling the surface of the pan and baking it in the oven for several hours prior to its first use. Thereafter, you cannot leave it in the sink, standing in water, or do an incomplete job of drying the surface. It will rust. Again, while cast iron is inexpensive and does a great job of cooking, it does require more attention to its care. It is not for everyone.

Copper is handsome, very expensive, and an excellent conductor of heat. It should be heavy gauge and lined with another metal. Because of its high cost, many manufacturers put copper only on the bottom of pots and pans. If you are paying copper prices, be sure that you are getting a sufficient layer of copper. What looks like copper bottoms is sometimes either a very thin veneer of copper or a less expensive copper-colored metal.

Teflon-coated cookware requires little or no fat for cooking and is easy to clean. Purchase good quality utensils. The cheaper Teflon finishes will scratch and wear off easily.

Most cookware is sold in sets, although pieces can be purchased individually. The sizes you will need depend on your family size. If you are cooking for three, you probably do not need a five-quart saucepan. The basics are three saucepans, one each of sizes 1 quart, 2 quart, and 3 quart; and one skillet either 8 or 10 inches in diameter.

Look for flat bottoms. The whole surface of the pan should be in contact with the heat source. Cookware that is too thin in construction will warp and no longer sit flat. Heavy ware spreads the heat more evenly to keep food from spot scorching and sticking.

Appliances

There are so many electrical appliances today that your kitchen countertops could begin to look like Mission Control at Cape Canaveral. Appliances require floor, counter, or storage space. They sometimes are not energy efficient, and sooner or later they will break down, requiring time, money, and maintenance.

Think twice before you invest. Will the appliance be used regularly? Does it have more than one use? Will the frequency of use justify the investment? Will it require special cleaning procedures which eat up your time after meals? (Sometimes appliances gain time for us on one end of the spectrum and rob it from us on the other end.)

Toaster vs. Toaster-Oven or Broiler-Oven vs. Microwave

You can almost guess when a couple was married by the type of toaster appliance they have. When my grandparents were married in 1918 they received a toaster which was set on a burner on the stove to toast. When my parents were married in 1943, they received three new electric toasters with fold-down sides. Cousins who married in the fifties and sixties received pop-up toasters. And today most brides receive toaster-ovens.

Toasters

A limited-purpose appliance may not be the best investment of your money or kitchen space. If you need a toaster just once daily to brown three slices of bread, you might consider another alternative. On the other hand, my grandmother had a toaster that did six slices of toast at a time. It barely did the job, since she had seventeen children of her own and raised six grandchildren and various other waifs.

Toaster-Ovens

For most of us, a dual-purpose appliance is a better investment. A toaster-oven can be used to toast, bake, and heat. It is a fuel saver since you do not have to heat the whole oven to bake one potato or heat one frozen dinner. It is not a good investment if you use it only to toast bread.

Broiler-Ovens

The broiler oven is larger, heavier, and more expensive than a toaster-oven. If your stove does not have a broiler and you frequently broil foods, for example, chicken and fish, it is a worthwhile investment. Again, it is a waste of fuel and counter space to use a broiler oven only to toast bread.

Microwaves

Microwave ovens are the new-age kitchen appliance. They do not toast or brown or broil. They thaw, heat, cook, and bake in magically less time than would be required for these tasks by conventional methods. No heat is applied in the process.

Microwaves are short-length, high-frequency waves which radiate through the food, agitating the molecules, causing the temperature of the food to rise. It cooks from the inside out rather than from the outside in as happens with conventional ovens. I call this method "nuking."

Microwave cooking works best for those foods with a high moisture content. As a matter of fact, they will not heat low or no moisture substances. That is why the food containers do not heat. Since no heat is applied and the moisture content of plastic is low, plastics do not melt in a microwave but will melt in a conventional oven.

When first introduced, there were some questions about the safety of some of the original models. Some were not well insulated and small amounts of microwaves did escape. These problems have been corrected. The federal government has set strict standards for microwave oven construction, including a requirement that doors have interlocks which prevent them from being opened when the oven is on to preclude accidental exposure to microwaves. As a precaution, manufacturers suggest that those with pacemakers to stimulate their heart rhythms should avoid contact with a microwave. For the rest of us, microwave ovens are safe.

They are, in my opinion, a gift for the busy home executive. Frozen meals can be thawed and reheated quickly by the boss or by any of her family subordinates. Fresh vegetables cook in minutes and are bright in color and deliciously crisp. Leftovers can be easily reheated for a snack or a light meal.

A friend in California calls his microwave his "bacon cooker" because he says it crisps bacon better than any skillet. He is a doctor and knows better than to eat bacon daily! However, he is also from Oklahoma and thinks that breakfast is incomplete without bacon.

One of the most important attributes of a microwave is that you can cook without adding fats or oils. Because foods are cooked from the inside out, you do not need to oil the pan to prevent sticking.

Electric Skillets, Electric Woks, and Slow Cookers

An electric skillet is not an essential appliance, unless you do not have enough burners to meet meal preparation needs. It is a versatile cooker which can be used to stew, steam, bake, roast, braise, and pop corn.

It can also be used for frying. I do not recommend frying foods since they add fats. However, if you are going to fry foods *occasionally* and you have an electric skillet, you might consider using it. The thermostat control allows evenly controlled, high temperatures for frying which may decrease the amount of fat absorbed into the food as it cooks. Generally, avoid frying foods.

Many people like to use electric skillets and woks and slow cookers during hot weather because they feel that they do not heat the kitchen up as much as burners do. They can be used to serve hot foods on a buffet and, with an extension cord, they can be carried into the backyard for meals outside during warm weather. Unless you use them regularly, they can clutter your cabinets and tie up cash.

Look for those with a removable thermostatic heat control and timer so that you can immerse the entire skillet or cooker in water to wash it. This will make them safe for children to wash. Also look for ones with heavy bottoms so they will not tip over.

Electric Woks

Oriental-style stir-fry cooking became the rage in the late seventies and everyone received a wok for Christmas—many of them electric. Stir-frying is an extremely healthy method of preparing vegetables. They are quick-cooked in a very small amount of oil and water, which seals in nutrients and leaves vegetables crisp and bright.

My wok is not electric but fits over my stove burner like those used in restaurants. We eat Oriental style foods weekly. Yet I do not feel that this is frequent enough to justify the cost of an electric wok whose purpose is limited to this style of cooking. My Asian friends use their woks much like I use a skillet, but I cannot get accustomed to using it for anything other than stir fry.

Stir-frying can be done in a traditional skillet as can many other Oriental dishes. It is not necessary to purchase a special cooking vessel to include this nutrition-retaining cooking method in your meals. If you do invest in a wok, I would recommend the stove-top variety. You can find them for as little as $15 including wok utensils. If you want to buy an electric wok, follow the guidelines for selecting an electric skillet.

Slow Cookers

Slow cookers were another Christmastime bonanza. Advertised as a boon to the busy wife, they cook dinner while you work or play. My father, who eats little or no meat, uses his slow cooker to cook pinto beans, the protein staple of his diet. It is an excellent appliance for this purpose.

The biggest objection which people have to including dried beans, peas, and lentils in their diets as a substitute for meats is the time required to cook them. With a slow cooker, you can put the beans or lentils in to cook and forget about them until hours later.

The crockery from which the majority of these cookers is made makes them efficient energy users. You need not worry that they will drain your electric bill.

Slow cookers also make excellent soups and stews—foods which we think taste better if eaten a day or two after cooking when the flavors have blended together. The major disadvantage to this cooking method is the loss of vitamins which are destroyed by heat. Long cooking can destroy part of the vitamin C and thiamine (vitamin B-1) which are soluble in water and destroyed by heat.

Pressure Cookers

The two biggest advantages of a pressure cooker are time and fuel. You can cook most things in a pressure cooker in two-thirds less time than is required by other methods. Pressure cooking preserves flavor and nutrients, tenderizes tougher cuts of meats, and reduces cooking time for otherwise time-consuming products like beans.

However, you can never be unconscious or half-witted when using a pressure cooker. Most cookers build up around fifteen pounds of steam pressure. Improper use can result in explosions and scalding injuries.

When I was little, Mother inadvertently drilled a round hole in the ceiling above our kitchen stove. She had failed to properly insert the rubber gasket in the lid, and the top blew off. It was just the right size for an air vent, so Daddy installed one in the hole.

Today's pressure cookers have safety features which Mother's lacked. All have air-vent cover locks which allow pressure to build only when the cover is closed properly, preventing the cover from being opened until pressure is safely reduced. A visual indicator, a little button which pops up, tells you when the cooker has reached full pressure. All models have pressure regulators which allow excess steam to escape. And all have over-pressure plugs which automatically release steam if the regulator vent pipe gets clogged.

Never buy a secondhand pressure cooker. Older models lack some safety features which are built in today. Follow directions EXACTLY and do not leave pressure cookers unattended. Pressure cooker accidents, which are rare, are like small, private airplane crashes: most occur as a result of operator error rather than machine failure.

Coffeepots

I hate instant coffee and most perked coffees. This is the one place where I step back from labor- and timesaving devices. I like a good strong cup (pot!) of French roast coffee, freshly ground and dripped in a Chemex pot. It is probably because I feel like a researcher again, hand pouring water through the filter paper like we did in the chemistry labs at Berkeley. Consequently every morning my husband and I lie in bed as the snooze alarm repeats its demand that we arise, and try to bribe one another into getting up to make the coffee. Usually the person with the weakest bladder loses.

However, if you like to catch just one more wink, an electric pot with a timer can be a blessing. My father, for all the years of my parents' marriage, carried Mother's coffee to bed for her each morning, peach that he is. As a child I remember many a cold morning when I could hear Daddy shivering in the kitchen as he put the coffee on to perk and then shuttled back and forth checking it until it was ready.

When they acquired an electric pot, his job was somewhat easier. He could make a quick dash to the kitchen to plug it in, and need not worry that it would boil down to syrup if he didn't turn it off. Ah! but the real luxury came when I gave him a simple timer. He could now make coffee the night before, it turned on automatically, and he made but one trip to fetch their first cup of coffee to bed.

Today, if he chose to do so, Daddy could have a portable coffeepot with a five-inch television set and a radio built in. It sounds like an invention from Charlie Chaplin's *Modern Times*! Daddy says of this newfangled pot, "Next thing you know, they'll make one that will drink the coffee for you too!"

Beaters, Blenders and Food Processors

Beaters

If you frequently bake cakes, make bread, and so forth, you may want to invest in an electric stand-mounted mixer. If you rarely do, you might be content with a hand-powered rotary beater or a handheld light-duty mixer. Look for one with a good handgrip, gears which mesh smoothly, strong straight shafts, and beaters which do not bump each other.

If the only thing you ever mix are martinis, then all you need is a swizzle stick. If you only mix eggs for omelets, then a wire whisk or a spring whisk will do the job. They take up little space, are easy to clean, and burn calories when used with vigor!

Blenders

Blenders are useful for pureeing, mixing, finely chopping small quantities of food, and blending. They work best with liquid or semiliquid foods. They are great tools for preparing health drinks from whole fruits or vegetables and for making your own baby foods from food which the family is eating. They can be used to crush ice in mixed drinks, and to make sauces, gravies, and dressings.

A blender is not an essential kitchen appliance. If selecting one, buy the simplest, least complicated model you can find.

You do not need twelve buttons with names which suggest that the blender does twelve functions. All a blender blade does is go around in a circle at either slow, medium, or fast speeds. The more complicated the machine, the more likely to break.

Select a model which comes apart for cleaning. That is, one in which the blade comes apart from the container. Also buy one with a container with easy-to-read markings on the blender jar. If a small jar attachment is offered, you might want to buy it for chopping nuts. Finally, choose one with a sturdy base so that it will not tip over easily.

Food Processors

Food processors are extremely handy helpers to have around. They can chop, mince, slice, grate, mix, blend, puree, and make pastries and doughs. They combine the attributes of an electric mixer and a blender. They work so quickly and efficiently that you will feel as if you have added a sauce chef to your kitchen to do all of your prep work!

I first encountered a forerunner of the food processor when completing my dietary internship at the University of California, Berkeley. I was assigned to work with the dietitians in the main campus cafeteria which served 16,000 meals daily. In the bowels of the basement, I watched in wonder as the vegetable prep man processed 500 pounds of potatoes in less than 15 minutes in a high-speed vertical cutter.

For the next few years I daydreamed about owning a miniature model of this massive stainless-steel cutter which stood almost as tall as me. The first small commercial models were introduced in the mid-seventies by a French manufacturer, Cuisinart. I was still a student and heartbroken to be unable to afford one. A friend I had helped at an earlier time gave me a gift of one. Periodically I still send him thank-you notes and postcards, asking, "Was there life before Cuisinart?"

A food processor can revolutionize your kitchen work. I can make a whole wheat crust mushroom-cheese pie from scratch to placing it in the oven in 6 minutes. When construction workers were remodeling my husband's office, I served them a Mexican tostado dinner which took less than 5 minutes to slice radishes, tomatoes, olives, and lettuce for toppings.

For people who complain that fresh fruits and vegetables take too long to slice or dice, the food processor is essential. It will not slice foods as expertly as will a skilled chef. However, there is no need to have perfectly sliced mushrooms if you are just going to cook them. And with practice, you can get a very attractive product.

The fact that the processor makes pastries and doughs is also an asset. I make large batches of healthy cookies to freeze for lunches and snacks. Nuts are chopped and cookie dough whipped up in minutes in the food processor. It will not liquify, grind coffee, or beat egg whites, tasks which a blender will perform.

When selecting a food processor, look for the same attributes as in a blender: limited number of buttons, durable heavy base, readable markings on the container, and ability to disassemble completely for washing. A large feeder tube is preferable to a small one. This will permit you to slice whole fruits and vegetables. For example, whole slices of fresh orange to be marinated in Marsala wine for dessert.

Juicers

Unless you own an orange orchard, fresh-squeezed juice is the most expensive kind of juice. To make one glass of juice requires 2–3 oranges. Medium-sized oranges are usually 3–4 to a pound. At prices of 49–89 cents per pound, a glass of juice from frozen concentrate is a better buy.

If you regularly drink carrot, celery, or other vegetable juices, a juicer might be a good buy for you. In terms of nutrients, it is better to eat the whole food than to drink only the juice. This will ensure an adequate intake of fiber—the pulp or stringy part of the food which is discarded when juice is made.

Salad Dryers

To me this is another indispensable kitchen item. Introduced several years ago from Europe, the salad dryer is a plastic bowl with an interior perforated bowl which spins to force water from your washed salad greens. I wash two heads of leafy lettuce at a time, spin them dry, and use the container to store them until needed.

These dryers range in price from $8 to $25. We eat more fresh green salads when the greens are ready to toss with a light dressing than we do when we have to wash greens each time we want a salad. An alternative is to wash lettuce leaves, shake them dry, and store them in plastic bags with a paper towel to absorb excess moisture or in a muslin bag.

Strippers, Parers, Choppers, and Graters

Like me, you may be mesmerized by late-night television commercials for devices that peel, pare, chop, core, grate, and shape vegetables in the speed of a blink of the eye. The experienced demonstrators of these gadgets are truly magicians because once you get yours in the mail you can never perform the same miracles.

I have yet to find a device that beats doing these tasks by hand. Friends are forever giving me gadgets. The most recent was a "stripper." You place a hard fruit or vegetable on a rotating spindle and a tiny blade in a movable arm does the peeling.

The stripper does not work much faster than an experienced cook using a manual paring knife or a swivel-blade peeler. Nor does it do a complete job. You still have to finish off tops and bottoms.

Peeling vegetables is a job that rarely needs to be done. The peels of most are not only edible but excellent sources of fiber. In some vegetables, like potatoes, nutrients are more concentrated near the peel than in the interior. Peeling reduces nutrient value. Instead, wash the surfaces thoroughly with a vegetable brush. Remove blemishes, scars, and eyes. Then cook. We were pleasantly surprised recently when an expensive and elegant Manhattan restaurant served whole cooked carrots still in their peel. Unstripped vegetables could become the next cooking rage.

Knives

There are six basic types of kitchen knives listed below. The first three will meet most of your recipe needs. The other three are optional. Their names and styles vary slightly by manufacturer. Prices vary greatly. Some cutlery has become an art form and is presented in boxes like fine silver and sold in jewelry stores.

The *paring knife* is used for small work, curling, paring, trimming, and coring. It is needed for preparing fresh fruits and vegetables.

The *chef's knife* is used for slicing and chopping. The shape of the blade allows you to pivot the point of the blade on the chopping surface and work the knife quickly up and down to chop. The blade tapers from the point to a width wider than the handle when they met. This allows your knuckles to clear the chopping surface.

Scalloped or serrated blade knives are used for slicing bread and soft fruits like peaches and soft vegetables like tomatoes. If you bake your own bread, you may also want a bread knife. Otherwise this blade will suffice on the rare occasions you need to slice breads.

For those who frequently include meats in their diet, a *carving knife* and *boning knife* will be useful. *Kitchen shears* are also helpful in separating poultry into parts.

Most professionals use stainless or carbon steel knives. They are a bit more expensive but they are easy to take care of and hold a sharp edge longer. They can be sharpened with a stone or sharpening steel. My husband is an expert at this. He likes to put on a show when he sharpens—sort of a Benihana's at home.

When buying knives, the metal of the blade should extend all the way through the handle and be fastened with rivets. Handles should fit your fingers for a firm grip to prevent slipping. In the long run, it is cheaper to buy a well-made knife that lasts than to replace it every few years. Put your dollar into good blades and not into fancy handles or ornamentations common on gift-packaged sets.

Do not store knives in a drawer, unless you store them in a covering sheath. It is dangerous and they will lose their sharpness from banging against other utensils. Store them in a slotted board or on a magnetic holder.

Electric carving knives were another Christmas craze. Every uncle, brother, and nephew who has received ties five years in a row is subject to receiving an electric carving knife as a gift.

Unless you have severe arthritis, they are not great economic investments. They are fine for slicing boned roasts and big-breasted turkeys, but they are useless for getting meat from around bones. They are expensive, use energy, and are noisy to boot. They also deprive you of the skill of carving.

The "Please-Don't-Tell-Me-That-You-Have-One-of-These" List

The nutritional quality of otherwise perfectly good foods can be destroyed by some cooking methods. Unfortunately, special cooking devices and appliances have been designed for these methods. If you own any of these, I recommend that you use them as flower planters. Do not cook with them!

A deep-fat frying device called a Fry-Baby was a popular Christmas gift several years ago. Its primary purpose was to fry doughnuts—a food which is not needed on a regular basis in the diet due to its high fat and sugar content. It could also be used to deep-fry otherwise perfectly sound foods like potatoes, vegetables (dipped in a batter to absorb more fat), and small pieces of meat.

Hot-dog cookers are high on this list. Over ¾ of the calories in hot dogs come from fat. For people concerned about food additives, they also contain nitrites and other preservatives and color and flavoring agents. If you cannot go to a baseball game without eating a hot dog, go ahead. But owning a device whose sole purpose is to cook wieners seems to me to be a poor investment of capital and a food habit not to be encouraged.

Bacon cookers, like hot-dog warmers, encourage undue amounts of fats and additives in the diet. BLTs and bacon and egg breakfasts should be periodic, not frequent, meals.

Two other appliances which have limited purposes are waffle irons and popcorn poppers. If your family eats waffles every weekend, a waffle iron is a worthwhile investment—granted that you serve them with a fruit covering rather than floating in syrup! Popcorn can be popped in a standard skillet. An electric popper is handy for use by children in their play area. Without butter and salt, popcorn is a great finger snack food.

Cupboard Checklist

Table 7.1 lists basic equipment and appliances needed. Depending on your menus and cooking style, the list can be expanded. The items listed will permit you to prepare all the menus included in this book.

DOING AHEAD

Many of the tasks which need to be performed in a kitchen are repetitive and could be done in advance and in bulk. In large food service operations, such as restaurants, cafeterias, and hospitals, much of the preparation is done ahead and in quantities beyond those needed for the immediate meal.

TABLE 7.1 BASIC EQUIPMENT AND APPLIANCES

Preparation

Mixing bowls, graduated from 3 cups to 4 quarts	Measuring cups for dry ingredients
Rubber or plastic spatula	Measuring cup for wet ingredients
Hand or small electric mixer	Measuring spoons
Cutting board	Colander and/or strainer
Swivel-blade peeler	Cutlery
Vegetable brush	Paring knife
Can and bottle opener	Chef's knife
Grater with assorted grating surfaces	Serrated knife
Salad dryer	Wire whisk

Top of Stove

Saucepans, covered	Utensils
2-quart	Slotted spoon
3-quart or second 2-quart	Wooden spoon
1-quart or smaller	Basting spoon
Covered skillet	Ladle
10- or 12-inch	Pancake turner
Large kettle/pot	Two-tined fork
4- or 5-quart	

Oven

Casserole dish, 2-quart	Roasting and baking pan
Cookie sheet	Wire cooling/baking rack
Muffin tin	Loaf pan

Appliances

Toaster oven
Microwave oven
Pressure cooker or slow cooker
Coffeepot
Food processor

For example, if you daily serve a tossed salad with a meal, you can wash and prepare the lettuce and other greens in bulk and store them until used. The best storage unit is a salad dryer or crisper which first spins the greens to remove water.

When preparing a food which can be frozen and reheated, double the recipe and freeze half of it. This will give you meals for nights when you do not feel like cooking or when you are away and family members are on kitchen duty. It also gives you ready meals for unexpected guests. Lasagne, stews, curries, quiche, soups, macaroni and cheese, casseroles, cookies, and many hors d'oeuvres freeze well.

I set aside Thursday evening for all advance food preparation. I shop and have all deliveries arrive on Thursday afternoon. One major meal for the weekend is prepared so that we minimize kitchen time during our weekend.

Things which I commonly do in advance:

1. Wash and clean salad greens
2. Prepare carrots, celery, radishes, and other finger-food vegetables
3. Make bulk batches of muffins or any other breads or cookies
4. Make double tuna salad mix
5. Prepare any hors d'oeuvres for expected guests in upcoming days
6. Pressure-cook 1 pound of beans for use in various recipes
7. Prepare one casserole or main dish for use over the weekend
8. Prepare salad dressings for week (stored in Grolsch beer bottles)
9. Reconstitute fruit juices

TIMING MEAL PREPARATION

One of the most difficult problems for many cooks is understanding how to schedule meal preparation so that all foods are ready on time and so that preparation takes minimum time. The key is learning to write a preparation schedule which segments out the tasks to be performed, estimates the time required for each, then orchestrates them to occur simultaneously.

This is an exaggerated and admittedly rare, but true, case. I was once amazed to observe a woman who prepared each item on her menu to completion before starting the next. She read down her menu and prepared things in the order they occurred. By the time she had completed whipping the cream for her dessert, her once fresh vegetables had wilted and turned gray, her entrée had dried out, and her salad was limp.

Here's how to organize meal preparation.

1. First look at your menu. Which item will take the longest to cook? Which ingredients in the menu are duplicated in more than one recipe? (For example, chopped onions. You can chop all of the onions needed at once.)

2. Write down estimated preparation and cooking times.
3. Now calculate backward to determine when preparation must start. And remember that several things can go simultaneously. The chicken can roast while the carrots are boiling. The salad can be tossed while the rest of dinner is cooking.

Let's look at two examples (tables 7.2 and 7.3).

TABLE 7.2 ORGANIZING MEAL PREPARATION #1

Step 1: Dinner Menu
Roasted chicken
Brown rice
Carrots and Brussels sprouts
Tossed salad
Baked apples

Step 2: Estimated Times

Menu Item	Preparation Time	Cooking Time
Chicken	3 min	1 hr
Apples	5 min	¾ hr
Rice	2 min	¾ hr
Carrots	5 min	10 min
Brussels sprouts	5 min	10 min
Tossed salad	Made ahead	
Total	20 min	1 hr

Step 3: Calculating Backward—Schedule for Dinner at 6:30

Time	Task
5:30	Wash chicken; place on baking rack in baking pan; dust with ground herbs and seasonings; bake at 350° F for 1 hr
5:33	Core the apples; place in a baking dish; stuff core hole with raisins
5:38	Scrub carrots and slice on diagonal
5:43	Measure rice and water into saucepan
5:45	Turn rice on to cook; place apples in oven to bake
5:45–6:15	TIME OUT! READ THE PAPER, HAVE A SMALL GLASS OF WINE, VISIT WITH THE CHILDREN, RELAX!
6:15	Put saucepan of water on to boil; trim Brussels sprouts
6:20	Put Brussels sprouts and carrots on to cook; toss salad with dressing
6:30	Place chicken on serving platter, surround with drained carrots and Brussels sprouts; put rice in serving bowl; remove apples from oven to cool; place food on table

Simple food, simply prepared, can be delicious and nourishing. This chicken dinner has no added salt, sugar, or fat. It includes a balance of those nutrients which are essential to good health and a distribution of calories which limits fat intake.

Fortunately, the simplest foods save the most time and are also often the most nutritious. For example, an apple pie takes much longer to prepare than applesauce. It contains more fat (in the pie crust) and sugar (in the filling) than applesauce. There is more cleanup to do when making apple pie. Applesauce takes longer to prepare than baked apples. It is higher in added sugar.

Look for ways to move from simple to simplest since they often are paralleled by progressively greater nutritional benefits.

Simple ⟶ Simpler ⟶ Simplest
Apple pie ⟶ Applesauce ⟶ Baked or raw apples
Good nutrition ⟶ Better nutrition ⟶ Best nutrition

Notice when time is actually being saved and when it is just being shifted to another time slot. We could have fried the chicken in the above dinner and saved some preparation time. However, frying creates greasy cleanup of stove top, walls, and counter. It also adds unnecessary calories. So once again, that which is simpler, roasting, saves time and is nutritionally more beneficial.

This entire meal could have been prepared in advance. When you arrived home, you could have put the chili in the microwave to reheat—followed by the corn-bread muffins; toss the salad and orange slices with the dressing (orange slices stored in jar), and serve. The fruit would probably even taste better after the flavors had mingled all day.

Any leftover chili can be frozen either as a batch or as single serving portions. The extra corn-bread muffins made by doubling the recipe can be used in lunches or frozen for future meals.

The key to elimination of last-minute chaos and hectic efforts to slap a meal on the table, is PLANNING. Restaurant chefs do not go into overload when food orders arrive in the kitchen. They view each menu item with its component parts and proceed in logical order to execute the dish. They perform all similar tasks simultaneously. If several dishes will need chopped onions, they estimate the quantity to be used and chop all of the onions at once. They do not chop each onion for each dish.

They prepare much of the food in advance. Sauces, salad dressings, desserts, salads, vegetable preparation, and breads are made during the day rather than at the time of service. They

TABLE 7.3 ORGANIZING MEAL PREPARATION #2

Step 1: Dinner Menu
Vegetarian chili
Hot corn bread
Tossed salad
 Orange slices
 Poppy seed dressing
Fresh peaches and blueberries

Step 2: Estimated Times

Menu Item	Preparation Time	Cooking Time
Chili	10 min	30 min
Corn bread	5 min	20 min
Tossed salad	Made ahead	
Orange slices	3 min	
Poppy seed dressing	5 min	
Peaches	5 min	
Blueberries	5 min	
Total	33 min	30 min

Step 3: Calculating Backward—Schedule for Dinner at 6:30

Time	Tasks
5:45	In food processor, chop onion and garlic then shred carrots; in saucepan assemble precooked beans (from previous night), onion, garlic, carrots, and canned crushed tomatoes, season with cumin and chili, simmer for 30 min
5:55	Using standard scratch recipe, first double it, and make corn bread and pour into muffin tins, set aside
6:00	Using standard recipe, prepare poppy seed dressing; make a double batch directly into a bottle or jar and store extra in bottle in refrigerator for future use
6:05	Peel and slice orange and toss in serving bowl with salad greens and dressing—refrigerate until serving time
6:10	Put corn bread in oven; peel and slice peaches; wash and destem blueberries; toss together and put in refrigerator to chill
6:20	Use this 10 min to make lunches or do prepreparation on foods for tomorrow
6:30	Serve dinner

prepare in bulk. What they do not use today will be used tomorrow or frozen for the future.

Chefs usually have assistants to help with preparation. The sauce chef prepares sauces and gravies and is immediately junior to the chef. The produce chef cleans and cuts all fresh vegetables and fruits. The baker makes all breads and desserts.

You may have noticed that mention has not been made about table setting and cleanup. Along with many of the tasks just listed above, these can be delegated to other members of the staff.

CLEANUP

Get it while its hot might be a good motto for the cleanup crew. The sooner a pot or dish is at least rinsed after use, the easier it will be to clean.

Pots and Pans

Have a dishpan or sink of hot sudsy water ready to soak cooking containers while you are preparing the meal. As you empty a cooking container and utensils onto the serving dishes, place the used containers in the sudsy water. Many items, if washed at that moment, for example pots in which vegetables were steamed, can be cleaned instantly and without effort. The same pot left on the stove until after dinner will have to be soaked and scrubbed to remove dried juices, gravies, and sauces.

Except for containers with baked-on food, you should be able to have all preparation pots, pans, and bowls either washed or loaded in the dishwasher as they are emptied onto serving dishes. This is a good job to delegate.

Meal Dishes

As used dishes are returned from the dining area, scrape and rinse them with hot water. Whether they are to be handwashed or dishwashed, this hot-water rinse will remove most surface refuse before it dries and will make both forms of washing easier and more efficient.

Do not pile dishes all over the countertop, creating confusion. Scrape and rinse then stack them. They will be ready for washing after dinner and the job will go much quicker because it is already partly organized.

If you have a dishwasher, place dishes directly in the racks after they are rinsed. There is no need to handle a dish twice— for example, no need to rinse and stack on the counter and then later handle again to load into the dishwasher. This will, of course, require that before dinner you make sure that clean dishes in the machine are removed. Another good job to delegate.

Guests at our dinner parties are always amazed that my kitchen does not fall into chaos during the evening. I do not allow tasks to pile up nor handle a kitchen task repeatedly when it can be finished in one stage. Efficient business executives never handle a piece of paper more than once. They either dictate a response immediately or assign it to someone for action. They do not repeatedly read a piece of paper and set it aside or toss it into unidentified piles.

Fast or Between-Meal Dishes

Wash as you go can apply to family meals which are eaten on the run. At breakfast time, instruct family members to rinse and load their used dishes into the dishwasher rather than leaving them in the sink where food scraps and debris will dry on them and be difficult and time-consuming to remove. For handwashing, again prepare a pan or sink of hot, sudsy water and ask everyone to either wash his or her own dishes and place them in the rack to dry or at least drop them into the sudsy water so that someone else can complete the task in swift time.

Dishes left to stand in the sink in water makes an excellent grow medium for molds, bacteria, and other germs. Since not all cookware and serving ware are impervious to these germs—that is, some are porous—it is wise to avoid leaving dirty dishes around. They will also attract ants, flies, and cockroaches—even in the best of neighborhoods!

My dream kitchen eliminates all cleanup problems. It is constructed of stainless steel throughout, with terrazzo tile floors which slant toward a large drain in the middle of the room. After dinner, you put the dishes back into the cupboards, close the door to the kitchen, and flip on a switch. The room becomes a giant dishwasher and everything, including stove and counters, is washed sparkling clean!

Until some bright structural engineers can figure out how to construct such a kitchen, I will remain in charge of cleanup. I do delegate the lion's share of this responsibility. Good character training for the children!

Delegation

Many of the tasks listed above can be delegated to other members of the "corporate staff." Like an executive chef, you should be in charge of scheduling, delegation, and supervision. You need not be responsible for all the "doing."

> This is a story about four people named Everybody, Somebody, Anybody, and Nobody. There was an important job to be done and Everybody was sure Somebody would do it. Anybody could have done it but Nobody did it. Somebody got angry about that because it was Everybody's job. Everybody thought Anybody could do it but Nobody realized that Everybody wouldn't do it. It ended up that Everybody blamed Somebody when Nobody did what Anybody could have done. (Anonymous)

All too often we women tend to think that it is easier to do it ourselves than to delegate it, supervise it, police it when it still isn't done, and finally redo it because it wasn't done to our standards.

This is not a productive management attitude. Think how low output would be if company managers held this point of view. Productivity would be limited to the work which they alone could do. Obviously, productivity is dependent upon delegation of tasks.

It is time, as master planner of family nutrition, to delegate the tasks and responsibilities which are required to produce meals that will nourish, satisfy, and please your family. This may require some staff training, and even some untraining and retraining.

I am a nutritionist, not a psychiatrist, but I do suspect that several of the following things are true and can be used to your advantage to get the job done.

First, it is my opinion that part of the demise of the family as a unit which functions coherently and nurtures us emotionally and spiritually as well as physically is a result of lack of participation and responsibility within the family. When everyone in the family shrugs and announces "Let Mom do it," there is trouble in paradise.

"Let Mom do it" says that what I want doesn't count. If I do try to help, it will not be welcomed. If I do try to help, I will probably make mistakes and Mom will be upset. Mom doesn't notice what I do when I do help, so I will use my time for something else.

When there is a general sense that it does not matter whether or not you make a contribution, you often choose not to. Children in such homes may feel like burdens. Deep down inside husbands may feel like male chauvinist pigs, forcing you into household chores which hinder your pursuit of career or other interests. And you may feel neglected, burdened, overworked, unappreciated, and generally pissed off!

The solution is to delegate. Create a team with you as team manager. For each task that needs to be done, find a doer. Be specific in your delegations . . . make specific requests and give specific directions. Everyone should know exactly what is expected of him or her.

For example, give your six-year-old son the job of setting the table for dinner. Instruct him in how to do that task. You may have to supervise him closely the first several times.

Skill is built on practice. Continued practice in the face of "not yet perfect" is based on incentive and reward. You cannot train your dog to do tricks if you do not continually reward it for getting the trick right. To teach your dog a complicated trick requires that you separate the trick into sequential parts and teach them to the dog in order. People learn in the same way.

Clearly state or demonstrate what is expected. Throwing the flatware on the table in the direction of the plates and hoping that they land in place does not meet the criteria. It may take your child many tries to remember that the fork goes on the left of the plate and the spoon and knife on the right. And it may require some reminding that in addition to location, neatness is required.

As supervisor, your job is to rule on how well tasks were or were not done. Be profuse with your praise, especially in initial training phases when your "staff" lacks confidence about the tasks. Be specific with praise. Tell your son that he did an especially neat job today and you notice that the flatware is all perfectly aligned with the plate and table edge.

One of the most difficult parts of training is consistency. You cannot accept a poor job one day and criticize it the next. Dogs do not learn tricks this way and neither do people. You must be continually alert to the standards which you have set and consistent in your expectations about meeting them.

If the job is not up to snuff, point it out. Be sure to criticize the job and not the doer. For example, don't tell your son what a klutz he is if the job is not tidy. Yelling "bad dog" at Rover when he doesn't get the trick right will do nothing to train him. Explain exactly what is wrong with the job and what needs to be done to correct it.

For simple tasks, the training phase will not last long. Soon your charges will recognize their own mistakes and correct them without your intervention. Your input and feedback will no longer be needed as frequently. However, praise is still needed occasionally. When guests comment on how attractive your dinner setting is, be sure to add that your son always sets the table.

Your goal is to have a smooth-running operation with the ability to function under usual as well as variant conditions. Football teams and the military are trained in this way.

The military's Standard Operating Procedures delineate the responsibilities and required steps for all tasks which must be performed in order for a unit to function. There is never any question about what or how things are to be done. You just look it up in the SOP. This permits any soldier to replace another in doing a task. It also ensures that in an emergency, everything will function as expected without error. There will be no running in circles, wringing one's hands, and wondering what to do.

Football teams spend weeks before the season practicing standard offensive plays and learning patterned defensive responses to potential plays by opponents. Their goal is to be a mechanical functioning unit which can respond automatically to any opposing team's plays.

Your family can be trained equally as well. Make a list of all the standard tasks which must be done. Delegate them. (My mother posted them on the refrigerator like Luther's proclamation on the church door.) Train the delegatee to perform the task.

Consistently oversee and acknowledge their work. Remember, you are the boss. There is no superior to thank you for your work. But a major responsibility of your job is to let your helpers know that their work is appreciated. It takes you far less time to thank your son for his excellent table setting job than it takes you to do it yourself.

8. Recycling and Refuse— Leftovers

A time-honored tradition is "waste not, want not." While we often espouse this adage, as a population group, we fail to follow it closely. A new branch of science was initiated in 1973 at the University of Arizona in Tucson: garbagology, the study of garbage. Its first published study revealed that on the average we toss more than $100 per year into our garbage cans. The study did not count food we flushed down our garbage disposals, fed to our pets, put in our compost piles, or spilled on the rug. Nine percent of the food we brought into the house was wasted.

Often we waste food for lack of a better idea about what to do with it. Or we simply forget it at the back of the refrigerator and when we finally discover it, it has changed from ½ cup of tuna casserole into a thriving metropolis of gray-green fuzz.

By contrast, manufacturers waste little of their resource inputs when manufacturing a product. The butcher business offers the best example. Nothing is wasted. Blood drained from the carcass on slaughter is used in blood sausage. Hooves and horns become fancy buttons. The head is served up as headcheese. Bones and cartilage are used to make gelatins and thickeners or in fertilizers as bone meal. The tongue is smoked or boiled for delicious deli service. Brains are scrambled and served up with eggs. The tail becomes oxtail soup. The stomach lining is sold as honeycomb tripe, a popular ethnic dish. Intestines are used as casings for spicy, aged sausages. Intestinal contents become fertilizers. Meat scraps feed our dogs and cats in fancy formula pet foods. And we wear the skins and hides to dinner as shoes, handbags, belts, and coats.

Butchers claim to use everything but the "oink." Following their example, some manufacturers have built entire secondary industries on their by-products. Oyster farms off the Chesapeake Bay grind leftover oyster shells for sale to cement manufacturers. The hulls and shells from almonds are ground and mixed with other ingredients for sale as cattle feed. Sodium bicarbonate, a by-product of fertilizer production, is sold to us as baking soda.

A classic tale is told about Henry Ford and the Model T. In the initial stages of his business, when capital to install a full-fledged manufacturing facility was limited, Ford Motor Company was a fabrication house primarily dependent upon outside manufacturers to supply component parts for cars.

The Model T was the "workingman's" car and, like the Volkswagen ("people's car"), retained the same design year after year. This allowed Mr. Ford to standardize his vendor supply orders for component parts.

One year Mr. Ford's order for engines asked that they be supplied in very special crates. As a matter of fact, the specifications for the crates were as specific as those for the engines. They were to be perfect cubes made of prime wood with no flaws and made to within one-sixteenth of an inch accuracy. Vendors were warned that if the crates were damaged in any way they would be returned unopened and payments would not be made.

Mr. Ford's controller thought him slightly mad, for the additional crate specifications increased the cost of the engines by $3 per crate. Further, Mr. Ford issued orders to his crews that no one except a crew of specially trained personnel, using specially padded tools, was to uncrate the engines. Mr. Ford himself supervised the first uncratings, warning that anyone who damaged a crate would be fired.

Mr. Ford then closed his expensive carpenters' shops. The crate sides became the floorboards for his Model Ts at a cost of 50 cents per car. From the savings he was able to expand production and increase cash reserves.

Mr. Ford went beyond making use of a scrap, he actually created leftovers for a specific use. You do this at home when you buy a larger roast than you need to ensure leftovers to make sandwiches for bag lunches.

Many recipes call for ingredients which you could serve as a separate menu item one night and use the leftovers as an ingredient for another. For example, corn bread or corn muffins are a tasty and welcome warm bread. Leftovers can be used for enchilada pie, stuffing for a chicken, or dried and crumbled for use as bread crumbs.

Cafeterias are often ingenious in serving leftovers in new ways. I once worked in a hospital in California which served a pudding which was a favorite of patients, visitors, and staff. Called "Princess Pudding," it might have better been named "Mystery Mush." For indeed, there was no "recipe" and each week the pudding was mysteriously concocted from leftover desserts. The cook would clear the dessert refrigerator of all leftover cakes, pies, puddings, canned and fresh fruits, mix them together, cover them all with a custard, and bake them. The result was truly one of the richest, most delicious, and mysterious of desserts—fit for a princess!

RECYCLING

Using leftovers saves time as well as money. The initial cooking time has been invested, and now you simply incorporate the leftovers into another dish. These reuses often take less time since you are reheating rather than actually cooking the ingredients.

Several examples are listed in table 8.1. They are by no means all inclusive or exhaustive. The majority of cookbooks are indexed by ingredient as well as by recipe name. Thus if you have leftover beets, you should be able to look through the index and find recipes which use beets as a primary or solo ingredient as well as recipes in which beets are incorporated.

We sometimes create leftovers or waste because we fail to involve our "consumers" in meal planning. Before introducing a new product to the market, manufacturers conduct extensive surveys to discover whether such a product will fill a need or whether a need can be created for the product. Next they produce samples of the product and invite consumer test panels to taste and evaluate it.

Then they select a small number of cities in which to test-market the product. Local advertisements announce the product. Coupons or "two-for" offers may be given to induce a first purchase. Market researchers study purchase and repurchase pat-

TABLE 8.1 USING LEFTOVERS

Chicken or Turkey
  Roasted for first meal
  Leftover slices
    Reheated in light gravy
    Wrapped around asparagus or broccoli spears as chicken or
      turkey divan
    Hot or cold sandwiches
  Chunks and broken pieces
    Sandwich salad with chopped celery and onion
    Luncheon salad with walnuts and raisins
    Chef's salad
    Any hot entrée which calls for chicken chunks
      Creamed in pastry shells or over toast points
      Tetrazzini over spaghetti
      Noodle casserole
      Curry
      Chow mein
      Enchilada filling
      Potpies

Spinach
  Fresh in salads
  Fresh cooked as leaves or chopped
  Leftovers
    Rolled into fish fillets for fish Florentine
    Stuffed into spinach crepes for brunch
    Creamed with onions
    Added to lasagne
    Light supper frittata
    Added to soups
    Spinach soufflé

Vegetables
  Served fresh the first meal
  Leftovers
    Marinated in oil and vinegar to serve as salad or to toss with
      salads
    Used as a main ingredient in a dish
      Broccoli or green beans in chicken-noodle casserole
      Potatoes in hot or cold potato salad
      Cream of asparagus soup
      Squash or pumpkin fritters
    Added to other dishes
      Kernel corn added to corn bread or fritters
      Peas added to rice

TABLE 8.1 USING LEFTOVERS (cont.)

Fruit
   Served fresh as handheld fruit or sliced
   Leftovers
      Tossed together as fruit salad with yogurt
      Cooked with prunes to make hot compote to serve over pancakes
      Overripe bananas become banana bread
      Mushy apples become applesauce, apple fritters, or grated for
         apple cookies or cake
      Soft plums become tart topping

terns as well as interview new users to measure product acceptability. Only if a product passes all of these trials, will a manufacturer then go into full-scale production and distribution.

We generally do not proceed with such precaution when introducing a new food or dish to the family. The result may be uneaten food when everyone announces "I don't like this." Food companies do not feel angry, hurt, or rejected when we don't like their products. They withdraw the product from the market, try to recoup their losses, and begin work on a new product to replace the just failed one.

Children are particularly hesitant about new and unusual foods and dishes. Before they have tasted it they may announce that they don't like it. It may be that the name sounds funny to them or that it smells or looks different. My experience is that they are more interested in tasting a new dish or food and will be more likely to accept it if they have participated in selecting or preparing the food.

While working as nutritionist with preschool children in a San Francisco day-care center, I noticed that many of them would not eat carrots. So the teacher and I planned a full day's activities around carrots. First, we "planted" some carrots by putting carrots with tops still attached in a box of sand. Then I read them a story about a little boy who planted and cared for carrot seeds until they grow. The children pulled the green tops from the sand and were gleeful to discover carrots.

Next we learned all the ways to cut carrots—sticks, dice, cubes, slices, grated. Then we tasted them raw in each of these forms and talked about how the flavor changed. Next we cooked and tasted each of these forms. Finally we made carrot cake. Every child in the group left an avid fan of carrots.

You need not go to this extreme, but a little involvement can go a long way to smooth the introduction of new dishes, recipes,

and foods. Snarled noses whining, "What's this stuff?" disappear when kids are in the kitchen helping to prepare new dishes.

STORAGE

Leftovers should be stored in airtight containers to prevent drying out, to limit absorption of other refrigerator odors, and to detour bacteria and mold spores from growing.

Some nutrient losses will occur over time. From the moment a food is harvested, nutrient loss begins. However, it is a very slow process. Physical losses occur when outer leaves are removed. Chemical losses occur due to exposure to air and enzyme activity within the food. Some nutrients, like vitamin C, are more fragile than others and can be leached out by cooking, and destroyed by air or heat. Therefore, it is important to store all food, whether leftover or fresh, properly. Foods which have been cooked will need to be reused quickly or frozen to prevent further nutrient loss.

Store leftover vegetables with a bit of the liquid in which they were originally cooked. Then if you want to reheat them, you can use the same liquid and avoid leaching out any further nutrients. I steam vegetables so there is no liquor. I most often reuse them in a light marinade as a cold vegetable to accompany lunch.

Various types of storage containers are available for purchase. I personally prefer old peanut butter and wide-mouthed mayonnaise jars to plastic containers. The contents of the container are clearly visible and the containers are easy to wash immaculately clean. They do not discolor over time nor absorb nor give off flavors. They seal tightly and they are free.

I do have three large plastic storage boxes for freezer cookies. Old coffee cans work but do not seal well enough to prevent freezer burns (drying out) over time. The cans also do not use space as efficiently as the rectangular boxes do.

When choosing a storage container, try to anticipate how the leftover will be reused. If a piece of chicken is going into a lunch box to be reheated in an office microwave, wrap it in plastic wrap since you cannot put aluminum foil in the microwave. If that same chicken is going into an office toaster-oven, wrap it in aluminum foil since the plastic wrap would melt in the oven. It is a waste of wraps to store in one and reheat in another and a wast of your time to handle the wrapping twice. Think ahead.

If you expect to reheat a small amount of food for a meal or snack the next day, put it directly into an appropriate container for reheating. There is no need to put it in a storage container for overnight and then transfer it to a heating vessel the next day. Save yourself a step and a dishwashing job.

The very smallest amount of leftovers can be used. If not as a meal component or as an ingredient in an upcoming recipe, then as part of distant future meals. A friend who is a caterer has a "stock box" in her freezer. When she has a cup or less of vegetables which are not going to be used, she tosses them into the airtight plastic container. When it is filled, she makes "garbage" soup, a rich, colorful, and delicious delight.

Corporate profits depend on minimizing waste. Everything except the "oink" must be used, reused, recycled, or sold—at a profit. Corporate managers cannot carelessly allow parts to rust or deteriorate from poor storage and lack of planning. Once a component is purchased, it is debited against the corporation's income. Its cost must be recovered at point of sale.

We can throw out money by the cupful faster than we can earn it by the hour unless we include "planned overs" in our food management scheme. Thrift is an old-fashioned virtue which in today's high cost of food can pay big dividends.

9. Marketing Your Product

Manufacturers have a different way of packing, presenting, and pushing their products. The contents may be simple talc powder or vegetable oil, yet it is presented as if it were gold dust or precious essence. They know that things which catch the eye, catch the pocketbook.

Because we serve food daily we may forget to "market" it, to present it in eye-catching ways. We may also neglect to change our packaging periodically. Manufacturers know that when the same old talc powder gets a new, updated container, suddenly sales go up.

Such can be the case at mealtime. An attractively set table with changing centerpieces and a revolving combination of menus can create the impression of goodness, wholesomeness, and abundance. The very same menu served without imagination—without supporting "props"—can look dull, uninteresting, and unappetizing.

Man does not live by bread alone. We are nurtured by the ambiance, the emotional setting, the charm and serenity with which a meal is served. Our appetites can be whetted or wilted by the setting alone.

Consultants who develop layouts, meal concepts, menu design, and interior decorations for restaurants know the importance of integration. A Big Mac would not be nearly as much fun to eat, oozing and dripping onto a white tablecloth with silver candles, as it is to eat in the bright orange and brown color theme of McDonald's. Crepes would taste far less exotic and delicious served in a ranch-style decor on pottery plates than they taste served in the red, white, and blue French country kitchen setting at New York's La Crepe.

SETTING A PRETTY TABLE

You may feel that you barely have enough time to put the milk carton and the cereal box on the table. It actually takes very little additional time to set a pretty table and serve beautiful food. What it does take is planning and habit.

Start by analyzing the dominant theme to be followed. Then plan in variations which will allow for flexibility in menu and serving style. Most American families enjoy a comfortable meal-time style with some formalities but somewhat lax rules. They reserve formal, elegant dining for very special occasions or for restaurant meals.

Next inventory table accessories. What do you have which could but are not being used? How can you use existing items or pieces to add variety to your table service? If you choose to add accessories, what could be added which would give you the largest number of alternative combinations?

Planning table presentations is like planning personal presentation. Your wardrobe contains things which can be mixed and matched to meet your mood and to adapt to your career and social needs. Your table accessories can do the same. Just because that two-pieced blue suit came as a unit does not mean that you should abstain from mixing and matching the pieces with other items in your closet. Similarly, table accessories and tablewares do not have to be rigidly kept in sets.

Relax and be creative. Being original is not important. If you are all thumbs with no green ones and could never make "something from nothing," then just copy. Look for ideas and inspiration in magazines, show windows, merchandise displays, and other people's homes.

Select a standard plan for your table that works. This will be the staple presentation. Change table covering and napkins periodically to add variety. Then occasionally toss in a theme meal with table set to match the mood. Use every resource that you have. Unused items are a wasted investment.

PLACES TO EAT

Night after night at the dinner table can get boring—even if the place mats change colors. So I sometimes serve dinner other places.

Tray tables always come out of the closet on New Year's Day. We gather around the TV set to watch the Rose Bowl Parade, the big games, and to eat our sandwiches made from the Eve's leftovers. For major televised news events, like election night returns, we also drag out the tray tables.

Middle Eastern and Japanese dinners are served at the coffee table. Everyone sits on the floor on pillows or cross-legged. We eat with our fingers and listen to belly dancing music. Or fumble with chopsticks while listening to the strains of a Japanese flute.

Outdoor meals are a favorite. In the summer we ask friends to join us for free concerts in Central Park. We bring a blanket to spread and carry our dinner in a huge basket—huge because our appetites seem always as large as the outdoors! A large terry-cloth beach towel in the middle of the blanket marks the "table," and we use fabric napkins that will not float away in the evening breeze.

Tailgates of station wagons are the ceremonial serving place for buffets before football games. Your family and friends stand around the "table," filling their plates while they armchair-coach the impending game.

I must confess that my husband and I like to have breakfast in bed. And I don't mean just a roll in bed for breakfast. We like to carry in a tray with coffee, fruit, and grainy breads and the morning paper. Quiet dinners for two can also be served from a large tray on the living-room floor in front of a crackling fire. Send the children to bed early!

COVERINGS

In addition to what is on the plate, what is under the plate offers the most options for variety. Color, texture, and shape can be manipulated to create various moods and feelings.

The colors in your tableware will direct choice in table-covering colors. If your dishes have delicate pink flowers on the border, they will be lost against a deep earthen orange table-cloth. Work with, not against, what you have.

Select several color themes which work with your tableware,

then mix and match. As you select and mix colors, ask yourself what mood is created. Yellows, oranges, and reds are warm and cheerful. Greens, blues, and violets are cool and restful. Brilliant, clear colors are gay; neutrals and pastels are soft and subtle. Contrasting colors are vibrant, while related colors are stately.

Use a dominant color theme with small amounts of other colors added for accent. Unless it is circus night and you want to get the family in the mood, do not give everyone a different colored place mat and napkin with uncoordinated dishes. You might risk indigestion from such a setting as well.

Notice that certain colors remind you of certain seasons. Deep browns and oranges for fall; fresh, pure yellows and pinks for spring. Colors traditionally are associated with countries. Red, white, and blue are American and French; green, white, and red are Mexican; and we think of shining black lacquer and deep indigo blue as Japanese. By rotating the color combinations which are used, we can travel through seasons and other countries.

Some table coverings trigger automatic associations. A red-checkered tablecloth with a candle dripping down the sides of its wine-bottle holder and we are in Italy. That same cloth with biscuits in a basket and beans in a slow cooker and we are headed for a square meal on the south forty.

Solid-colored tablecloths give a sense of formality—even when they are in bright rather than muted colors. Thank goodness they are made today of soil-resistant, permanent-press fabrics. If they are not, consider using them rarely and sending them to a laundry.

One of my favorite tablecloths was a bed sheet. It was a gay blue and green pattern, perfect for buffets and outdoor meals. Absorbent terry-cloth bath cloths in bright red are carried in our picnic basket for cleaning up hands after finger foods. Bath cloths make great napkins for children.

Place mats decrease table setting time and are easier to care for than tablecloths. They come in vinyl and plastic materials which can be wiped clean rather than laundered. They can be quickly changed from meal to meal. They can be more easily mixed and matched with napkins to change mood.

Paper goods for the table once came in white only. We can now buy paper table covers and matching dishes in every color under the rainbow and in every imaginable pattern from pictures of Superman to Pilgrims and turkeys.

I personally rarely use paper goods—including paper napkins.

I like trees. Cloth and plastics are durable and will last for years. They also feel and look nicer than paper.

CENTERPIECES

Anything and everything from a silver vase to a fishbowl to a milk bucket or cookie jar can be used to hold flowers, fruits, leaves, or other greenery, or vegetables for a centerpiece. Remember that soup tureen that is gathering dust on the cabinet top? Fill it with autumn leaves. Sugar bowls, vegetable dishes, pitchers, and teapots can all become centerpieces. Let your imagination go. And be alert to ideas.

Nature is a brilliant artist and a great teacher. Take mental pictures of what you see in nature and store them for later reference. Note combinations of color, shapes, and types of plants. Jacqueline Onassis revolutionized centerpiece decorating at the White House when she had florists make relaxed, informal, mixed floral arrangements which mimicked nature.

Potted plants, with or without flowers, make simple and lovely tables. Use your cactus plants for Western dinners, your amaryllis bulb's first bloom for Eastertime meals, and English ivy when you are serving a simple Cheddar soup with dark bread and ale.

Use unconventional items. Your husband's or son's hobby model sailing boat flanked by used champagne corks and red and white streamers could announce a vacation. Children's musical instruments mixed with balloons and ribbons make a birthday or New Year's Eve theme. A miniature robot or spaceman surrounded by flags celebrates launch day for the first woman into space.

Some things become tradition. I have a little orange, ghost-shaped candle that Mother gave me at Halloween when I was in college. It is part of every All Souls Day table setting. Square candles covered with whipped paraffin and sparkles, a gift from friends at Christmas, are always part of the holiday decor.

Baskets can be used for flower, vegetable, or fruit arrangements. They can even be used for serving foods—raw vegetables, sandwiches, fruit, and cookies look inviting enough for Little Red Riding Hood's granny when offered in a basket with a bright cloth.

LIGHTING

Lighting contributes to mood as much as centerpieces do. Bright lights and bright colors encourage activity and conversation.

Fast-food operations which want their clientele to enjoy and leave quickly, use this principle. Restaurants which expect you to linger over a meal, relaxed and unhurried, use dim, unobtrusive lighting and subdued colors.

We have a dimmer in the dining room. It works like a volume control. As we turn the lights down, guests lower their voices! Unfortunately this trick is lost on children! They always want to know why we are whispering.

Candles make an elegant and romantic mood. Even your most basic lasagne seems richer and fuller in flavor when served by the flicker of candlelight.

FOOD PRESENTATION

A Swedish friend invited us to dinner, promising to introduce us to her native foods. We were thrilled and arrived with properly starved appetites. Hors d'oeuvres were a smoked fish in sour cream and onion on water crackers. The soup course was a cream of oyster served with dainty white rolls. When the main course arrived, our eyes experienced white-out fatigue! Butterfish with new potatoes and cauliflower served on bone china.

We eat with our eyes as well as with our noses and our mouths. An all-white meal is excruciatingly boring. As is one in which fish occurs three times, two courses have cream in them, and all textures are smooth and soft. A bit of attention to variety in color, texture, and shapes of foods adds tremendously to a meal's appeal.

Restaurants garnish plates with parsley and orange slices to improve the appearance of their food. Food editors spend hours laboring over arrangements of foods for photographs for their magazine pages. Manufacturers have "suggested serving" photographs printed on their labels which include colorful additions to enhance the appearance of their product. All know that pretty food sells.

Color influences our perception of taste. A green cake will only sell on Saint Patrick's Day and blue foods don't sell at all. We do not think that they will taste good. Never mind that color has no taste. We act as if it does! Hospitals and other institutional food services put red food coloring in lemon Jell-O when they are out of raspberry and strawberry flavored because red sells better. If you ask a customer who has just eaten this Jell-O what flavor it is, he or she may well respond, "red."

In part our visual reaction may be learned. We have learned that vegetables which are gray from overcooking are less crisp and delicious than vegetables which are bright in color. We have learned that fruits which are brown are overly soft and mushy instead of juicy and fresh.

On seeing a mountain of white rice piled high on a platter, our eyes prepare us for a different gastric experience than when we see rice with bits of chopped red tomato, glistening yellow onion, and green parsley. Before we put a spoonful in our mouths, our eyes have signaled a report to our taste center and we prepare for the expected.

My friend's endless white dinner was like a blizzard. After a bit, you could no longer see. Our eyes were signaling our taste buds that we were doomed to sameness. While the tastes of each component of her meal were quite distinct, we could not tell. Still no amount of parsley could have saved the meal.

My father-in-law, a lover of food, is an advocate of parsley and other garnishes. He believes that the simplest and least expensive meal, presented with attention and care, can be a feast for kings. And right he is! A cream soup with a sprig of parsley or a dash of paprika or a few chopped chives on top looks more inviting than a plain cup. Croutons, shredded cheese, a lemon slice, and chopped olives also liven up a soup. It looks like you cared.

Foods cut into unusual shapes add interest. A peanut butter sandwich cut into quarters and arranged in a pinwheel looks tastier than an unsliced one. The same old vegetables cut into numerous shapes appear to be different foods. Carrots and other hard vegetables can be curls, rounds, cubes, sticks, crinkle-cut, or cut on the diagonal. They actually do taste a little different when cooked due to the change in surface area.

Pay attention to the arrangement of food on the plate when serving it, even if you serve it family style and fill the plates at the table. Foods in overlapping piles in the center of the plate look as if they were slapped on by the cook's helper in a military field operation.

When I was little I was fanatical about my foods not touching. I wailed if foods were piled together and would not eat parts that "touched." There was no explanation for this fanaticism. There is no need to strictly separate foods, but they do look better if they are distinguishable.

A last idiosyncrasy: Serve sauces and gravies on the side rather than poured over the food. First, this allows everyone to take as little or as much as he or she likes. More importantly, it allows your diners to see what they are eating. Children are particularly suspicious of "mystery" foods and will hesitate to eat things that they do not recognize. No need to disguise a piece of fish with so much sauce that it is not visible.

Our sense of sight is critical to our enjoyment of a meal. We truly do taste with our eyes first. We often next sniff before we sample. Our noses tell us whether we can expect to taste tart, sweet, spicy, pungent, musky, oily, or herby.

A popular children's game asks blindfolded players to identify tastes when their noses are being presented with a smell other than that of the food they are actually tasting. An orange tastes like a lemon when the player is smelling a lemon. A wedge of peach tastes like a strawberry when the player is smelling a strawberry.

Manufacturers spend millions of dollars annually to discover chemicals which will reproduce taste and smell sensations. They are so skilled at their art that some unfortunately curious people drank a liquid dish detergent that smelled like the freshest and juiciest of lemons. It smelled too edible to be soap.

When we do finally put a spoonful of food into our mouths, we have two simultaneous experiences: the first actual taste of the food and a reaction to its texture. We notice whether the food is crisp, grainy, smooth, rough, soft, hard, liquidy, dry, spongy, soggy, and so forth.

Children seem to have more opinions about texture than adults do and may have food preferences based on texture alone. Jennifer loves raw carrots but hates cooked ones, especially if they are "mushy." You have all met children who will not eat their ice cream until it has been stirred round and round in the bowl, missing the sides and dripping on the floor, your new carpet, and their new clothes, and melted thoroughly. They then lick it off the spoon.

Variety in textures in the meal makes it seem as if there is more food. If all three items in a meal are mushy, you have no sense of change and everything seems like everything else. If there is one crisp, one mushy, and one grainy food, the meal seems more abundant although there are still only three items.

WHAT YOU CALL IT

The worlds of advertising and marketing have much to teach us about presentation and sales. When we read an advertisement that states, "Pango Peach color by Revlon comes from east of the sun . . . west of the moon where each tomorrow dawns . . . is succulent on your lips and sizzling on your finger tips and so will be one's own adventure in paradise," we are ready to buy.

Now we know, deep down inside, that Pango Peach was made in some laboratory in New Jersey, not east of the sun or anyplace near where tomorrow dawns. And we know that succulent and sizzling adventures do not happen at 9930 Fourth Street, no matter what color our nail polish. But it sounds great and it sells.

Begin to notice the names which manufacturers and restaurants give to their food products. "Country-style Vegetables with Chicken" conjures up a warm, brick-walled kitchen with pots bubbling on the burners and children with freckles playing in the corner.

But what are "country-style" vegetables? Where my folks come from that means rutabaga, turnips, and greens. They would be disappointed to buy this product and find that "country-style" means carrots, potatoes, and onions. To them that is Yankee food, not country.

"Suprêmes de Volaille a l'Ecossaise" is the same old chicken and vegetables in French. "Escargot" means snail. God knows we would never eat them if they were called "snails." It reminds us of those creatures who are forever invading our gardens!

When the family asks, "What's for dinner?" your reply can make or break the meal ahead. Tuna noodle casserole is descriptive but not exciting. Noodles Romano with Tuna sounds far more interesting. An omelet sounds tastier than scrambled eggs. Pâté sounds better than ground chicken liver. Hawaiian Ham sounds more intriguing than ham with pineapple chunks.

I sometimes write out menus for each person for special dinners. The foods do not have to be difficult to prepare or serve. But the names do need flair. For a Chinese New Year's dinner, I copied the dish names in Chinese characters on parchment paper and rolled and tied them like scrolls for each guest. The dishes were standard, inexpensive Chinese foods, but they seemed fancier when introduced to guests in this way.

Children love creative and festive food names. A pork and beans, biscuits, salad, and cookie meal for a group of boys can be introduced as Cowboy Beans, Hardtacks, Greens, and Chewers. The same meal for your teenage daughter's French study group could be called Cassoulet, Croûtes, Salade, and Galettes.

If you think that your family pays no attention to these details and that they will "eat anything," no matter what its presentation, think again. It may be that their senses have been so blunted by repetitive, bland, and boring meals that they no longer look forward to or expect things to be otherwise.

It takes no more time to prepare a colorful meal with contrast in texture and flavors than it takes to prepare a dull meal. What it does take is planning and attention to detail. Haphazard, unplanned meals give the impression that they took little time to prepare. Well-planned meals present an impression of goodness, wholeness, and abundance. They look as if great time and effort were put into them.

10. Market Trends

To survive in the marketplace, corporations must keep up with trends in consumer preferences, life-style, and economic changes, and shifts in response to their product. Corporate executives continually seek information on factors which might influence the acceptance and profitability of their products.

This information is so critical that several of the most financially successful businesses in the United States are companies devoted to analyzing and tracking trends. Yankelovich Skelly and White, Market Research Corporation, Food Marketing Institute, A. C. Nielsen, and Consumers Union are among the leaders reporting on food trends.

Like doctors, these companies are pulse takers. They monitor and report on the health of the nation's economy, family disposable incomes, spending and borrowing patterns, purchasing preferences, points of purchase, employment patterns among women, and hundreds of factors which affect what we buy, when and where we buy it, and how much we are willing to spend for it.

As chief executive officer of your own productive entity, you must take the pulse of your own population. Two factors are foremost in monitoring your family. First the family is not stagnant. It is an ever-evolving, ever-changing unit.

As the family ages, family roles change, individual family member needs change, preferences change, and so forth. The family is always in flux. The family never just "is." Families change so fast today that the minute the words are spoken to characterize it, the description is outdated.

This is easily apparent when our children are small. One day your son can barely crawl, and the next day, without warning, he stands and walks. At that moment, he no longer "is" the infant that he was before. And in the very next moment, he will again change.

We have a tendency to become stuck in our perceptions of our family. We even say things like "Susie never eats beets," which may have been true when Susie was three. However, since we have not offered beets to Susie since then, we do not know whether it is still true when Susie is thirteen. She may never eat beets only because they are never served.

We continue to cook what was once our family's favorite foods, without noticing whether or not they are still favorites. Family members have food experiences outside of the home where they are introduced to new concepts which may markedly change their preferences. A good example is the child who leaves for camp, a devoted hot-dog junkie, and returns announcing that he is now a vegetarian. Usually changes are unspoken and more subtle. If we are not sensitive to and looking for these changes, we will continue to serve fried chicken and gravy to a family which would really prefer skinless chicken baked with herbs.

Second, the family does not exist in a vacuum. Families exist in a social environment where each individual is impacted by what other individuals and families do, think, prefer, have, and offer. Truly, no man is an island.

Your task then is not only to be conscious and alert to changes within your family, but also to recognize trends in our social environment which flavor their food preferences. It would be nice to hire the Naisbitt Group (author of *MegaTrends*) to make reports to you. Unfortunately, only the largest of corporations can afford their excellent reporting service.

However, the information gathered by these trend watchers is available to you. As a matter of fact, the information is you. It is what you do, what you see, what you value. You need only to become more aware of how you and your environment are changing.

FASHIONABLE FOODS

Food styles, like cars, clothes, and furniture styles, change. One year everyone is eating fondue, soufflés, and quiche. The next, no real man would eat quiche, and the rest of us are nibbling stir fry, pasta, and tofu.

Dancer Fitzgerald Sample, a New York advertising agency, publishes *New Product News*, which reported that 2000 new food products were introduced in 1982. Many of these products were low-calorie, low-salt, or low-fat. Three major canners, Libby's, Del Monte and Hunt-Wesson Foods, introduced entire lines of no-salt or low-salt products in 1982.

The year 1982 also saw the introduction of caffeine-free products. Seven-Up, Pepsi, Dr Pepper, and Royal Crown Cola all rushed to enter this market. In the same year, all added aspartame, a new artificial sweetener (see page 34), to their low-calorie beverages. We spend over $10 billion annually on soft drinks while the percentage of diet drinks is growing at the rate of 11–12 percent per year.

"Lite" and "light" have become words that sell, not just to women. Low-calorie beers are marketed at least as heavily to men as to women. Calorie-controlled frozen dinners and entrées are advertised in men's magazines. They too have become weight conscious and the food industry is responding to their new awareness.

"Health" foods, once available exclusively in health food stores, are now sold by mainstream grocers. The words "natural," "whole," "wholesome," "hearty," "earthy," "unprocessed," "additive-free," and "no preservatives" sell. No longer are these foods made exclusively by people living in communes on the California coastline. The "generals," General Mills, General Foods, and General Nutrition Corporation, are making them in Minneapolis, White Plains, and Pittsburgh.

"Gourmet" also sells. Croissants have moved from small French bakeries to the kitchens of Sara Lee and Pepperidge Farms. Spaghetti sauce, once a staple made by Chef Boyardee, must now be Paul Newman's gourmet-style. The words "TV dinners" will no longer sell sliced roast beef in gravy with potatoes and peas. But the same dinner, with a gourmet label, is marketable.

Even popcorn has gone gourmet. In 1968 we ate 333 million pounds of popcorn. In 1983 we popped over 618 million pounds into our mouths. Much of the increased sales were from new gourmet popcorn shops where you can buy popcorn in as many flavors as you can buy ice cream.

"Exotic" fruits and vegetables are finding their way onto our plates. Peas and green beans will no longer suffice. We must now offer our family and guests a choice of various bean and alfalfa sprouts, bok choy, celeriac, chayote, daikon, enoki mushrooms, fennel, ginger root, jicama, kohlrabi, nopales, salsify, snow peas, sunchokes, spaghetti squash, and tomatillos. And for dessert, they can choose among cherimoya, guava, kiwi, lychee, mango, papaya, persimmon, plantain, pomegranate, prickly pear, quince, sapote and ugli fruits.

We once worried about what bars our husbands might be frequenting. We need no longer worry. They are drinking far less hard liquor than at any time in the past and have switched to wine and beer. Further, the bar which they are sidling up to is the sushi bar, the salad bar, or the health bar.

Fast-food marketers across the country are lightening up their menus. In 1979, Wendy's International introduced the first salad bar in a fast-food operation. Other burger vendors immediately followed their successful lead. This year Wendy's will introduce nationally its "light side" menu offering salad and sandwich entrées with less than 300 calories.

Restaurants in major cities across the nation are offering low-calorie meals to their customers. The hamburger patty, peach half, and cottage cheese plate is being replaced by deliciously prepared and interesting entrées. For example, The Four Seasons Restaurant in New York City, world renowned for its fabulous and rich food, offers Spa Cuisine for its weight-conscious clientele.

The original owner of Wendy's sold his interest and opened the first chain of "semihealthy" fast-food establishments called D'Lites which is based in Atlanta. With fast-food operations coming on strong in the low-calories arena, can it be long before we have "McSprouts," a salad in a sandwich from McDonald's?

Eating out is on the rise. The National Restaurant Association estimated that we spent $37.3 billion on fast foods in 1983, an increase of 5.7 percent over 1982. The fastest growing category of fast foods is Mexican, followed closely by chicken.

Attracting us to the fast-food counters involves big bucks in advertising. In 1982, $578.1 million was spent to advertise fast foods. The advertising budgets of the three top fast-food vendors paid off in sales (table 10.1).

TABLE 10.1 ADVERTISING BUDGETS OF FAST-FOOD VENDORS

Company	Advertising (Costs in Millions)	Sales (Millions)
McDonald's	$161.1	$6362.0
Burger King	65.1	2191.4
Kentucky Fried	42.6	1700.0

SPOTTING TRENDS

While it is difficult to quantify trends, it is not difficult to spot them. When everyone took to skateboards and roller skates, you could not help but get in their path on sidewalks. When Boy George and Elton John sunglasses came into vogue, you could no longer find large Jackie O. shades. Nehru jackets and bell-bottom pants are so passe that used-clothing stores do not even have them.

Three years ago kids chewed Flintstone vitamins. Today they prefer to eat E.T. Barbie is a has-been, replaced by Cabbage Patch Kids, Rainbow Bright, and Strawberry Shortcake. The Brady Bunch is boring. And the Jackson Five have come alive again with Michael. If you cannot locate your vacuum cleaner, check your children's room. It is probably strapped on one of their backs as part of a Ghostbusters' getup.

RIDING THE SHIRTTAILS OF TREND SETTERS

Marketing personnel are expert at appealing to our every motivation, interest, and desire. They both create and copy trends. Their techniques and technology can help us to promote better nutrition among our family members.

Marketers know that a basic personality quality present in each of us to some degree is competitiveness. We want to keep up with the Joneses. If the Joneses serve snow peas with water chestnuts and almonds at their dinner parties, you are not going to serve that green bean casserole with canned soup and canned onion rings at yours.

Pay attention to what your family members' peer groups are doing. If Johnny Jones eats gremlin-shaped chocolates for his snack, your daughter will want them too. Instead, offer them "gremlin cakes." Mix nuts, raisins, seeds, peanut butter, and oatmeal and pat them into little cakes. Perfect for gobbling up whole. Or invite them to put cheese on a slice of whole wheat bread and put it in the microwave to watch it bubble and spurt just like an exploding gremlin.

We desperately want to belong to the group and to do what the group does. If this is "the beer beer drinkers drink" then you can bet that those who consider themselves to be beer drinkers will drink it. If the Pepsi generation is alive and having fun, we will join it by drinking Pepsi, whether or not we are having fun!

During the 1984 Olympics you could have fed your family anything offered at the training table and they would have loved it. In the deepest recesses of their hearts, they each dreamed about being a member of the pavilion crowd. When the trumpets sounded, they visualized themselves walking onto the stadium field with Mary Lou Retton, the gold medal winner in gymnastics.

We want to be skillful and able and will eat foods which we believe will give us those qualities. If Juliet Prowse dances better because she drinks prune juice, then the ballet student at your house will drink prune juice in the hope of dancing better. When marathon runners began carbohydrate loading, you could for the first time feed your family tons of pasta without one complaint.

Advertisers use endorsements by respected authorities and famous names to promote their products. "Abe Lincoln" molasses is not an old family business handed down to today. Neither is "George Washington" corn chowder. They are respected old names used to sell new goods.

When Vincent Price tells us which brandy he prefers, we are likely to select it over its competitors. After all, he knows quality food and beverages. The most recent and clever use of recognized names is the introduction of several spin-off products from the television series, *Dynasty*. A new perfume, Krystle, a line of dressy clothing called Dynasty Collection, and a sugar-free dry beverage mix, also called "Crystal Light" have just been introduced.

We all know that Michael Jackson does not drink and Brooke Shields does not smoke. We know that Sylvester Stallone cautiously watched his diet to make weight for *Rocky III* and that he tutored John Travolta through the same route for *Staying Alive*. These are facts that can be used to encourage your family. Point them out. Invite your family to join these stars in their quests. Match Michael's abstinence, top Travolta's weight loss, or stay up with Stallone's mileage.

SUCCEEDING

You see, it is all the same old stuff in new packages. Dr. Mark Hegsted, a world-renowned nutritionist from Harvard University Medical School, says that our nutrient needs have changed very little over time. Certainly, we are engaged in less physical work and therefore need fewer calories for this aspect of our lives. We are perhaps confronted with more stress and strain in daily living, and this may slightly alter our nutrient needs. We are certainly confronted with more pollutants—noise, air, water—than in our past.

But the net effect of all of these changes is small. The Recommended Dietary Allowances are reviewed every three to five years. Changes are made when and if the eminent nutrition scientists who review them feel that our nutrient needs have altered significantly. They also comment when they feel that our food supply has changed in any regard, positively or adversely.

They have made no dramatic or drastic changes in the RDA. Our food supply is both abundant and wholesome. If we select foods properly we can provide more than the number of nutrients which we need from foods readily available. And if we avoid or use in moderation those food products which threaten increased risks of disease, we will be slim, trim, and healthy.

Succeeding with family nutrition is not a new game. The elements of success are the same as in any other pursuit.

Elements of Successful Nutrition

Commitment to Your Goal

We sometimes call this determination or drive. It is that quality which helps us to steer our grocery cart away from the aisles filled with cookies, cakes, and other goodies, knowing that they cost us cash and calories. They are off-purpose purchases.

When we are committed, we have a plan of action to implement or express and reflect our commitment. Thus, we have menu plans which meet our family's nutrient needs. We have budgets which reflect our spending needs and capacity. We have standard operating procedures for meal preparation, presentation, and cleanup.

Success does not occur by caveat or chaos. It occurs by plan.

Alertness

When we are asleep at the wheel, unwanted and unneeded foods creep into our grocery carts, bulging our budgets and bikinis. It is when we are least conscious that we stuff ourselves with extra mouthfuls of food. We wake up, moaning, "I can't believe I ate the whole thing!"

Shopping lists remind us of what food items we need for the meals planned. The list is like a road map stirring us down only those aisles which have foods we plan to use. Serving foods in controlled portion sizes helps us eat enough but not too much.

Success does not occur by osmosis during mindless moments. It occurs when we are alert and in command.

Attention to Details

When we plop spinach noodles and broccoli on the same green plate our appetites plummet. When we serve lemon and oil dressing on our salad, lemon sauce on the fish, and lemon sherbet for dessert, our tastebuds sour.

Meals which are colorful, have variety in taste, texture, flavors, and aromas, are hits with all audiences. The most basic of ingredients, offered in simple dishes with garnish and flair, get rave reviews.

Success does not occur by accident. It occurs when we are thoughtful of little things.

Lee Iacocca does not arrive at his office every day with "hope" that his products will sell and that his business will be profit making. He arrives every day with a commitment to producing a car that functions properly, is stylish, requires minimum upkeep and maintenance, and has an affordable price.

Your family will not be well nourished from "hope." But they will be well nourished, healthy, and excited about family food if you become the committed chief officer of nutrition in your household and begin to run your kitchen like the corporate entity that it is.

I invite you to tackle it. Take it on like a joy and a game to be played with your family. Make them your board of directors as well as your most responsible staff members. Enjoy it and enjoy the good health and good feelings which will result. My very sincerest best wishes to you.

Appendix

MANAGEMENT WORK SHEETS

To help you get started, following are blank forms for you to use in planning menus, preparing a shopping list, and establishing an inventory system. The steps are easy.

MENU PLANNING
1. Select one of the three patterns, whichever is most similar to the way your family currently eats.
2. Write in the foods you will use for each meal.
3. For serving portion size, check the item in the food group lists which follow the menu blanks.

TABLE A.1 PATTERN I: 3 MEALS AND 1 SNACK

Food Groups:	Dairy	Protein	Fruit	Vegetables	Carbohydrates	Fats and Oils
			1600–1800 Calories			
Breakfast	1	0	1	0	1	0
Lunch	1	1	2	2	2	0
Dinner	0	2	0	2	2	0
Snack	1	0	1	0	1	1
Total	3	3	4	4	6	2
			2200–2400 Calories			
Breakfast	1	0	2	0	2	1
Lunch	2	2	2	2	2	0
Dinner	0	2	0	3	3	2
Snack	1	0	1	0	1	1
Total	4	4	5	5	8	4

TABLE A.2 MEAL PLANNING BLANK

Meal/Group	1600–1800	2200–2400	Food Item to Be Eaten
Breakfast			
Dairy	1	1	
Fruit	1	2	
Carbohydrate	1	2	
Fat and oil	1	1	
Lunch			
Dairy	1	2	
Protein	1	2	
Fruit	2	2	
Vegetables	2	2	
Carbohydrate	2	2	
Dinner			
Protein	2	2	
Fruit	0	2	
Vegetables	2	3	
Carbohydrate	2	3	
Fat and oil	0	2	
Snack			
Dairy	1	1	
Fruit	1	1	
Carbohydrate	1	1	
Fat and oil	1	1	

TABLE A.3 PATTERN II: 3 MEALS AND 2 SNACKS

Food Groups:	Dairy	Protein	Fruit	Vege-tables	Carbo-hydrates	Fats and Oils
1600–1800 Calories						
Breakfast	0	1	1	0	2	1
Lunch	1	0	1	0	1	0
Dinner	0	2	0	2	2	1
Snack I	1	0	1	2	1	0
Snack II	1	0	1	0	0	0
Total	3	3	4	4	6	2
2200–2400 Calories						
Breakfast	1	1	1	0	2	1
Lunch	1	1	2	1	2	1
Dinner	0	2	0	2	3	2
Snack I	1	0	1	2	1	0
Snack II	1	0	1	0	0	0
Total	4	4	5	5	8	4

TABLE A.4 MENU PLANNING BLANK

Meal/Group	1600–1800	2200–2400	Food Item to Be Eaten
Breakfast			
Dairy	0	1	
Protein	1	1	
Fruit	1	1	
Carbohydrate	2	2	
Fat and oil	1	1	
Lunch			
Dairy	1	1	
Protein	0	1	
Fruit	1	2	
Vegetables	1	2	
Carbohydrate	1	2	
Fat and oil	0	1	
Dinner			
Protein	2	2	
Vegetables	2	3	
Carbohydrate	2	3	
Fat and oil	1	2	
Snack I			
Dairy	1	1	
Fruit	1	1	
Vegetables	2	2	
Carbohydrate	1	1	
Snack II			
Dairy	1	1	
Fruit	1	1	

TABLE A.5   PATTERN III: 2 MEALS AND 3 SNACKS

Food Groups:	Dairy	Protein	Fruit	Vege-tables	Carbo-hydrates	Fats and Oils
			1600–1800 Calories			
A.M. Snack	1	0	0	0	1	0
Lunch	1	1	0	2	1	1
P.M. Snack	1	0	1	0	0	0
Dinner	0	2	1	2	2	1
Night Snack	0	0	2	0	1	0
Total	3	3	4	4	5	2
			2200–2400 Calories			
A.M. Snack	1	0	0	0	2	0
Lunch	1	1	0	2	2	1
P.M. Snack	1	0	1	0	0	0
Dinner	1	2	0	3	2	1
Night Snack	0	2	2	0	1	0
Total	4	5	3	5	7	2

TABLE A.6   MENU PLANNING BLANK

Meal/Group	1600–1800	2200–2400	Food Item to Be Eaten
A.M. Snack			
Dairy	1	1	
Carbohydrates	1	2	
Lunch			
Dairy	1	1	
Protein	1	1	
Vegetables	2	2	
Carbohydrates	1	2	
Fat and oil	1	1	
P.M. Snack			
Dairy	1	1	
Fruit	1	1	
Dinner			
Dairy	0	1	
Protein	2	2	
Fruit	0	1	
Vegetables	2	3	
Carbohydrates	2	2	
Fat and oil	1	1	
Night Snack			
Protein	0	1	
Fruit	2	2	
Carbohydrates	1	1	

FOOD GROUPS

Following are the food groups to be used in planning menus and in determining serving size. Remember, if you are watching your waist, pay particular attention to serving size. Extra ½ teaspoons of butter can add calories fast.

TABLE A.7 DAIRY FOODS GROUP
(Approximately 100 Calories)

1½ cups skim milk
1 cup low-fat milk
¾ cup whole milk
1 cup low-fat buttermilk
1 cup low-fat plain yogurt
1½ slices (1½ oz) cheese

TABLE A.8 FRUIT GROUP
(Approximately 50 Calories)

1 small apple, orange,[a] pear	1 medium peach, fig, tangerine[a]
2 medium plums, apricots, prunes, dates	⅓ cup cranberry, apple, pineapple juice
¼ cup prune juice, grape juice, apricot nectar	½ cup orange juice[a], grapefruit juice[a]
½ cup pineapple, canned in its own juice	1 cup peaches, canned in water or own juice
½ small banana, grapefruit[a]	¼ cantaloupe, honeydew
10 cherries	12 grapes
1 cup watermelon, raspberries, strawberries	½ cup fruit cocktail, canned in water or natural juice
2 tbsp raisins	⅔ cup blueberries

[a] Vitamin C rich fruits.

TABLE A.9 VEGETABLE GROUP
(Approximately 40 Calories)

½ Cup Raw or Cooked

Artichoke hearts	Green beans
Asparagus	Kale
Bean sprouts	Onions
Beets	Sauerkraut (rinsed)
Broccoli	Tomato juice (unsalted)
Carrots	Tomatoes
Collard greens	Turnips
Eggplant	Wax beans

1 Cup Raw or Cooked

Beet greens	Mushrooms
Cabbage	½ cup cooked spinach
Cauliflower	2 cups raw spinach
Cucumbers	⅓ cup tomato sauce
Green bell peppers	Summer squash and zucchini

Unlimited Amounts

Celery	Radishes
Lettuce	

TABLE A.10 PROTEIN FOODS GROUP
(Approximately 150 Calories)

2 oz cooked *lean* beef (hamburger, steak)
2 oz cooked *lean* pork (1 small chop)
2 oz cooked *lean* chicken without skin (1½ legs, ½ whole breast)
3½ oz tuna (packed in water)
4 oz shrimp
3 oz cod, haddock
5 oz sole, scrod
2 eggs (watch out: 250 mg cholesterol each . . . limit weekly intake)
½ cup cottage cheese (cut calories by using low-fat)
¾ cup cooked dried beans or peas
1½ tbsp peanut butter (less 1 fat allowance)
1½ oz cheese such as Cheddar, American, Gruyère, Swiss, Muenster, Jack, Parmesan

TABLE A.11 CARBOHYDRATE FOODS GROUP
(Approximately 75 Calories)

1 slice bread, whole grain or enriched
1 small dinner roll or biscuit
½ hard roll, hamburger or hot-dog bun, English muffin, bagel
½ medium or 1 small potato, baked or boiled . . . PLAIN
1 small or ½ medium muffin—corn, blueberry, bran
1½ cups popcorn (NO butter or salt!)
1 cube (1½ in. square) corn bread
1 tortilla, 6 in.
1 slice pizza crust (¼ of 10-in. pie)
½ cup cooked cereal, farina, oats, grits, wheat meal
¼ cup granola (high in sugar)
½ cup whole grain brown or white enriched rice, cooked
½ cup cooked whole grain or enriched noodles, macaroni, spaghetti
2 3-in. griddle cakes
5 2-in. square crackers
1 6-in. whole wheat or enriched pita (pocket) bread

TABLE A.12 FATS AND OILS
(Approximately 100 Calories)

1 tsp butter
1 tsp mayonnaise
1 tsp margarine
2 tbsp gravy
2 tbsp cream sauce
1 tbsp heavy cream (sweet or sour)

1 tsp vegetable oil
2 tbsp salad dressing
⅛ of 4-in. avocado
2 tsp cream cheese
6 small nuts: almonds, cashews, filberts, etc.

TABLE A.13 TREATS
(Approximately 150 Calories)

½ cup ice cream	1 small serving French fried
½ cup frozen yogurt	potatoes
¾ cup ice milk	2 small cookies
5 oz (½ typical serving)	1 brownie
milk shake	1 slice cake
1 cup hot chocolate	1 doughnut
1 small serving onion rings	½ cup pudding or Jell-O
	1 oz trail mix

CHECKLIST

Corporations have quality assurance divisions which check to see if products are up to snuff. When you have completed your menus, check the following:

1. Among the fruits and vegetables planned, is there
   A very good vitamin C source?
   A very good vitamin A source?
   A dark green leafy vegetable?
   At least one serving which is raw?
2. Among the carbohydrate foods planned, are they
   Predominantly whole grain products?
   Some enriched or fortified products?
   Few highly processed, refined products (crackers, sugary cereals)?
3. Among the dairy foods, are
   Most selected in low-fat or skim versions?
   Extra servings included for pregnant and lactating women?
4. Among the protein foods, is there
   At least one meatless meal weekly?
   Only lean, trimmed beef or pork or skinless poultry
   Fish at least one meal weekly?
   No fried, only broiled, baked, or poached recipes?
5. Is there variety in color, texture, flavor, and aroma?

SHOPPING LIST

From the menus planned, you are now ready to prepare a shopping list. If you have a running inventory checklist, such as that below, some of your shopping list will already be completed.

Group foods on your list in the order in which they occur at the grocer's where you shop. This sounds like an unnecessary step but it will save you hundreds of steps and time when you do not have to return to aisles for items which you overlooked on your list when you first walked past.

Staples: Nonperishable

nonfat dry milk	canned milk	whole wheat flour
baking powder and soda	cornmeal	tuna, water-packed
wheat garm and bran	honey and molasses	pastas, several types
rice	canned tomato paste	canned tomatoes and sauce
beans, lentils, etc.	popcorn	canned clams
oil, safflower and olive	vinegar: cider and wine	peanut butter
spices and seasonings	raisins	sunflower seeds
walnuts	almonds	bread crumbs
oatmeal	cornstarch	soy sauce and tamari sauce
sesame oil	sherry wine	unflavored gelatin
olives	tea	extracts, vanilla, almond

Staples: Perishable

fresh milk	potatoes	yogurt
cottage cheese	juices	breads, at least two types for sandwiches
cheese	fresh vegetables	
frozen pastry shells	frozen spinach	fresh fruits
frozen peas	tortillas	onions and garlic

Menu Supplies (write in your own)

DELEGATION

I mentioned that my mother posted our weekly work tasks (she was from Texas so she called them "chores") on the refrigerator. Here is a sample of my family's chart. It leaves little doubt about who has to do what, when. We are flexible and do take one another's jobs. And Steven and I do attempt to get the other to make coffee even when it is our turn!

The "score" at the right of the page is our rating system. It is a very flat system. You either did the job well or you did not. There is no "sort of" or "half" scores. A sandwich with just mayonnaise on it is really not a sandwich. A table without the napkins is not set and a kitchen without the stove wiped clean after cooking is not a complete job.

Scores are X for complete and O for incomplete. There is no incentive, that is no reward money, for doing your job. But it is rewarding for us all to see a row of Xs at the end of the week and know that we got the job done!

Your chart will fit your family's needs, time schedules, level of skill, life-style, and so forth. A couple of comments about ours. I prepare breakfast because my office is at home and I do not have to commute to school or work in the morning. When Jennifer is with us, she cleans up after she dresses and eats and while she is waiting to leave for day school.

Jennifer prepares and cleans up her afternoon snack because she is the only one who eats one. When I join her, we share this task.

Weekend dinners are free-for-alls as indicated by the F. We all pitch in depending on what each of us is involved in for the day. Remember that one main dish for the weekend is prepared on Thursday night, so unless we have guests for dinner, there is not a lot to do over the weekend.

I also do most of the dinner cooking. Again, Steven commutes while I have to walk from my office to the kitchen, a distance of several hundred feet. I enjoy cooking and cook as a hobby. So for me it is not a burden.

Set up your own schedule so that it supports your career and activity commitments and your own level of (or lack of) joy in cooking. A nutritionist friend of mine who has very long work hours and a commute does little of her family's cooking. Her husband works closer to home and thereby has inherited this job. Another friend who actively volunteers at a hospital in her community leaves most of the cooking to her teenage sons.

Steven does cook when I am up against publishing deadlines or when television scripts need memorizing or when he needs a creative outlet. He is by nature a brilliant cook and also enjoys the kitchen.

Do not forget to delegate shopping chores as well. Teenagers are great shoppers and often have a free afternoon (when grocery stores are less busy) to do this task. Like husbands, they too can be asked to pick up specialty goods like fresh fish if a market is on their route home.

TABLE A.14 SAMPLE
FAMILY MEAL FLOW CHART—WEEK I

Meal/task	Member/Day							
	Mon	Tues	Wed	Thurs	Fri	Sat	Sun	Score
Breakfast								
Make coffee	A	S	S	S	S	A	A	
Set table	A	S	S	S	S	J	J	
Cook and serve food	A	A	A	A	A	A	A	
Clear table	J	J	J	J	J	J	J	
Stack washer	J	J	J	J	J	J	J	
Lunches								
Sandwiches	A	A	A	A	A	A	A	
Fruit	J	J	J	J	J	J	J	
Vegetables	A	A	A	A	A	A	A	
P.M. Snack								
Prepare	J	J	J	J	J	J	J	
Clean up	J	J	J	J	J	J	J	
Dinner								
Salad preparation	S	S	S	S	S	F	F	
Vegetable preparation	A	A	A	A	A	F	F	
Entrée	A	A	A	A	A	F	F	
Bread and butter	J	J	J	J	J	F	F	
Set table	J	J	J	J	J	F	F	
Wash pots as you go	S	S	S	S	S	F	F	
Clear and rinse dishes	J	J	J	J	J	F	F	
Clear condiments, etc.	J	J	J	J	J	F	F	
Stack washer	A	A	A	A	A	F	F	
Clean kitchen	S	S	S	S	S	F	F	
Garbage out	J	J	J	J	J	F	F	

TABLE A.15 FAMILY MEAL FLOW CHART

Meal/Task	Member/Day							
	Mon	Tues	Wed	Thurs	Fri	Sat	Sun	Score
Breakfast								
Make coffee								
Set table								
Cook and serve food								
Clear table								
Stack washer								
Lunches								
Sandwiches								
Fruit								
Vegetables								
P.M. Snack								
Prepare								
Clean up								
Dinner								
Salad preparation								
Vegetable preparation								
Entrée								
Bread and butter								
Set table								
Wash pots as you go								
Clear and rinse dishes								
Clear condiments, etc.								
Stack washer								
Clean kitchen								
Garbage out								

Index

Acutane, 54
additives, food, 63, 201–3
adults, ideal weight for, 83, 89–90
advertisements:
  on calcium deficiency, 62–63
  eating out and, 254–55
  fear of cooking encouraged by, 200
  food labels and, 26
  of hair analysis, 66
  new products and, 79
  special sales in, 159
aging:
  calcium intake and, 62–63
  metabolic rate in, 94
  physical activity in, 63, 88, 94
  vitamin E and, 55
  weight gain in, 87–88
Agriculture Department, U.S., 21
  on animal-protein consumption,
    114–15
  canned and frozen produce as
    graded by, 170
  dietary guidelines of, 28
  grading of produce by, 167–68
  on national sugar intake, 29–30
  on weekly food costs, 156
Agriculture Extension Services, 167

alcohol, 39–40, 41
  changes in intake of, 253, 254
  dining out and, 140
  low-calorie, 253
American Cancer Society, 38
American Heart Association, 28, 38,
  51
American Spice Trade Association,
  152
amino acids, 41–42
anemia, iron deficiency, 68
appliances, kitchen, 213–20
  see also equipment, kitchen; specific
    types
arachidonic acid, 47
arsenic, 59
artificial sweeteners, 33–34
ascorbic acid (vitamin C), 56–57, 76
  iron absorption and, 69
aspartame, 33, 34, 253
atherosclerotic diseases, 49

bacon cookers, 223
baking:
  diet margarine in, 150
  fats and oils in, 149
  sugar in, 152–53

barley, 181–82
basal metabolism, 23
beans, 194–95
  recipes for, 195
Beard, James, 153
beaters, 218
beef, beef products:
  commercially prepared, 190–92
  cooking, 150–51
  quality grades of, 187–88
  see also protein foods group
Benoit, Joan, 85
beverages, in thermos containers, 134–
  135
birth control devices, iron loss and,
  68
"Blahs," sugar intake and, 31–32
blenders, 218–19
blood sugar, 92–93
body fat, 46–47
body frames, weight and, 82–83
bone meal, 64
boning knives, 222
Bread Pies, 147
breads, 133, 182–83
  food labels on, 182
  fruit, 183
  refined white flour in, 182
breakfast:
  skipping, 93–94
  sugary foods for, 31–32
Briggs, George, 203
broiler-ovens, 213, 214
budget:
  inflation and, 155
  nutrition and consideration of,
    22
  weekly food costs in, 155–57
  see also costs, comparative
bulgur, 181–82
bulk purchases, 160
  of dry goods, 208–9
  of produce, 167
butter, 48
  margarine vs., 179

cadmium, 59
caffeine-free products, 253

cakes:
  fat in, 149
  purchasing, 187
calcium, 62–65, 77
  daily supplement of, 64
  excessive intake of, 64–65
  sources of, 63
calories:
  burned in daily activities (table),
    98
  burned in exercise (table), 97
  in carbohydrates, 36
  energy measured by, 23
  in fat, 36, 49–50
  portion sizes and, 103
  per pound of body fat, 47
  in protein, 36
  sources of, 91–93
cancer:
  fat intake and, 51
  fiber foods and, 37
  nitrites and, 189
  oat bran and, 185
  selenium and, 66–67
  vegetables and, 106
  vitamin A and, 54
  zinc and, 65
canned milk, 177–78
canned produce, 170–75
  brands of, 170–71
  cost of, 174
  grades of, 170–71
  nutritional drawbacks of, 171–74
  salt in, 174–75
  sugar in, 174
carbohydrate foods group, 107–8,
  265
  purchasing items in, 181–87
carbohydrates, 29–40
  alcohol and, 39–40, 41
  as cellulose, 29
  chemical composition of, 29
  complex, 29, 34–39
  diets low in, 34, 35–36
  fiber and, 36, 37–39
  refined vs. unrefined, 107–8, 182
  simple, 29–34
  as staple food, 29
  as starches, 29, 34–37

thiamine and intake of, 57
see specific types
cardiovascular diseases, 49
Carolyn (crisis eater), 142–44
carotene, 54
Carver, George Washington,
    196
carving knives, 222
cast iron cookware, 212
cellulose, 29, 37–38
centerpieces, 245
cereals, 185
cheese, 133
    imitation, 180
    natural, 179, 181
    processed, 180
    purchasing, 179–80
chef's knives, 221–22
Child, Julia, 153
children:
    creative food names and, 249–50
    ideal weight for, 84
    market trends and, 251–58
    school lunch programs, 136
    snacking by, 130–31
    "toddler" foods for, 122
    whimsical preferences of, 238–39
chloride, 59–60
chocolate milk, 177
choice grade meats, 188
cholesterol, 49–51
    atherosclerosis and, 49
    blood levels of, 50
    cooking methods and, 151
    egg substitutes and, 193–94
    manufacture of, 50
    purpose of, 49
    sources of (table), 52
Claiborne, Craig, 153
cleanup, 229–33
    of cookware, 229
    delegating responsibilities, 231–33
    dishwashers and, 229–30
    fast or between-meal dishes and,
        230
    fried foods and, 227
    of meal dishes, 229–30
    training phase in, 232–33
cobalamin (vitamin B-12), 58, 77

cobalt, 59
coffee, in thermos containers, 134–
    135
coffeepots, 217–18
commitment, successful nutrition
    and, 258
complex carbohydrates, *see* starch
    foods
congestive heart failure, 61
Consumers Union, 251
convenience foods, 197–201
    advertisements of, 200
    cost of, 198–200
    nutrition in, 199
    time saved by, 198, 199–200
convenience stores, 161–62
cooking, 148–53
    cholesterol in, 151
    dairy products in, 149–50
    fats and oils in, 148–49
    meat in, 150–51
    nutritional quality destroyed in,
        222–23
    poultry in, 150–51
    salt in, 151–52
    spices in, 152
    stir-fry, 216
    sugar in, 152–53
costs, comparative, 135
    of animal-protein sources, 113–14
    of beef, 188
    of butter and margarine, 179
    of cheeses, 180
    of coffees, 134
    of convenience foods, 198–200
    of crackers, 184
    delivery services and, 161
    of eggs, 193
    of fake foods, 197
    in food budgets, 155
    of imitation milk products, 176–77
    of juices, 164–65
    of peaches (table), 174
    of peas (table), 171
    of pork, 188
    of potatoes, 186
    of school lunches, 136
    of spices, 152
    of treats, 187

costs (*cont.*)
    in "twofer" sales, 163
    unit pricing and, 162–63
    of yogurts, 178
cottage cheese, cooking with, 149–
    150
couscous, 182
crackers, 184
Cuisinart, 219
cyclamate, 33, 34

dairy foods group, 104, 263
    in cooking, 149–50
    imitation, 176–77
    low-fat products in, 149–50
    purchasing supplies from, 176–81
Dancer Fitzgerald Sample, 79, 253
deficiency diseases, 23, 27, 79
delegation of responsibility, 209, 231–
    233, 267–70
    flow chart for, 269–70
delicatessens, 161–62
delivery services, 161
Del Monte, new products of, 175, 253
densitometry, 85–86
"Depression Della's Dinners," 145–
    147
diabetics, 33–34
diets, weight-reducing:
    brown-bag lunches in, 137
    celebrity endorsements of, 256
    complex carbohydrates emphasized
        in, 36–37
    "dieter's plates" in, 138
    "fabulous fructose" claims in, 33
    fast foods and, 138
    fiber in, 38
    fruit portions in, 105
    low-carbohydrate, 34, 35–36
    lunches, 137–40
    physical activity vs., 95
    portion control in, 103
    pregnancy and, 120
    protein tissues burned in, 42
    self-diagnosed hypoglycemia and, 32
    skipping meals in, 93–94
    snacks in, 111, 131
    trends and, 253, 254, 256
    very-low-calorie, 95

dinner:
    eating out, *see* restaurant meals
    as single daily meal, 93–94
dishwashers, 229–30
D'Lites, 254
dolomite, 64
Dynasty, products associated with,
    256

Eastern Market (Washington, D.C.),
    167
eating habits, U.S.:
    animal protein in, 43–44, 114–15
    cholesterol in, 51
    complex carbohydrates in, 36
    dining out in, 254
    fiber in, 38
    food budget in, 155–57
    health problems related to, *see*
        health risks
    meat in, 43–44
    protein in, 40–44
    salt in, 61–62
    sugar in, 29–30, 31
    sugar substitutes in, 33–34
    surveys of, 21–22
    vegetables in, 105–6
    waste in, 234
eating patterns, personal, 91–95
    calorie needs in, 101–2
    distractions in, 130
    portion size in, 103
    regularity in, 130
    small, infrequent meals in, 93
    snacking in, 129–32
    sources of calories in, 91–93
    three types of, 101, 110–11
eggs, 192–93
egg salad, "mock," 150
egg substitutes, 193–94
electric carving knives, 222
electric skillets, 215–16
electric woks, 215–16
electrolytes, 59–61
    loss of, 61
Equal, 34
equipment, kitchen, 210–23
    beaters, 218
    blenders, 218–19

broiler-ovens, 213, 214
checklist of, 223, 224
coffeepots, 217–18
food processors, 219–20
juicers, 220
knives, 221–22
microwave ovens, 213, 214–15
pots and pans, 211–13
pressure cookers, 216–17
salad dryers, 220–21
slow cookers, 216
toaster-ovens, 213–14
toasters, 213
versatility in, 210–11
exercise, 95–99
aging and, 63, 88, 94
appetite reduced by, 96
calories burned after, 95–96
calories burned by types of (table),
97
calories burned daily by (table),
98
cholesterol levels and, 51
dieting vs., 95
electrolyte loss in, 61
energy required by (table), 97
muscle weight and, 83–85
osteoporosis and, 63
scheduling, 98
two types of, 98

family life:
changing nature of, 251–52
chores shared in, 231–33
delegation of responsibility in, 209,
231–33, 267–70
social setting of, 252, 255–56
farmers' markets, 167
fast foods, 138
advertisement of, 254–55
"light," 254
fat cells, total of, 94
fats, 46–51
caloric intake and, 36, 49–50
cancer and, 51
chemical composition of, 47–48
in dairy foods, 104
dietary need for, 47
diseases related to, 49, 51

energy provided by, 46
in meats, 188, 189
protein intake and, 42, 44, 45, 107
reducing intake of, 148–49
sources of, 48–49, 52
types of, 48
unsaturated, 48
vitamin E and, 56
fats and oils group, 108, 109, 265
carbohydrates and, 107–8
in cooking, 148–49
nonstick cooking sprays vs., 149
fiber, 36, 37–39, 220
excessive intake of, 38–39
types of, 37, 38
in unrefined vs. refined products,
107–8
fish, 192
flatulence, beans and, 194
flours, refined white, 182
fluoride, 70–71, 78
folic acid (folacin, folate), 58, 77
pregnancy and, 120
Food and Drug Administration, U.S.
(FDA), 26, 34, 202
food labels, 26–27
on breads, 182
on commercially prepared meat
products, 190
"dietetic," 175
on fake food, 202
fats and, 48–49
on juices, 164
order of ingredients on, 30–31
salt on, 62
sugar on, 30
Food Marketing Institute, 251
food processors, 219–20
Ford, Henry, 17–19
floorboards ordered by, 200, 235
Four Seasons Restaurant (New York,
N.Y.), 254
freezing foods:
advance food preparation and, 224–
225
fish, 192
leftovers, 240
French Market (New Orleans, La.),
167

Friedman, Milton, 205
frozen foods:
    fish, 192
    grades of, 170
    salt in, 174–75
    "squeeze" test for, 161
fructose, 32–33
fruit breads, 183
fruit group, 104–5, 164–75, 263
fruits:
    appearance of, 168
    bulk purchases of, 167
    canned, 170–75
    "exotic," 254
    frozen, 170–75
    grading of, 167–68
    hints for selection of, 168
    leftover, 238
    locally grown, 166–67
    in lunches, 135
    in produce terminals, 167
    with sauce or gravy, 175
    seasonal availability of, 170, 171–
        173
    storage of, 168
    treats vs., 104–5, 109, 170
"fruit sodas," 166
Fry-Babies, 223
frying foods, 148, 216
    cleanup after, 227

garbagology, 234
generic brands, 170–71
goiter, 69
good grade meats, 188
"gourmet" food trends, 253
graters, 221
gravies, 149
    ready-made, 175
    served on side, 247–48
gums (fiber), 37, 38

hair analysis, 66
Health and Human Services
        Department, U.S., 28
Health and Nutrition Examination
        Survey (HANES), 21–22, 87
"health" foods, 253

health risks:
    alcohol intake and, 40
    artificial sweeteners and, 33
    cholesterol and, 49–51
    excessive intake of food and, 22,
        27–28
    fats and, 49, 51
    hypertension and, 60–61
Hegsted, Mark, 257
hematocrit, 68
hemicellulose, 37–38
hemoglobin measure, 68
herbs, cooking with, 152
high density lipoprotein (HDL), 40,
        50–51
honey, 32
hot-dog cookers, 223
Huevos Rancheros, 145
Hunt-Wesson Foods, 253
hydrostatic weighing, 85–86
hypertension, 60–61
hypoglycemia, 32

infant feeding, 121–22
    seasonings in, 122
    solid foods in, 121
    table foods in, 121–22
insulin, 92, 93
iodine, 69–70, 78
iron, 67–69, 78
    pregnancy and, 68, 120
    vitamin C and, 69
Italian Meals (contingency plan),
        145–46

juicers, 220

kidney stones, 64–65
King, Alan, 56
kitchen management, 15–20
    chief executive officer in, 17–18
    components in, 22
    dream vs. reality of, 17
    elements of, 18–19
    excellence in, 20
    goals defined in, 18
    objections to, 15–17
    objectives in, 21–22

plan of action in, 18–19
poorly vs. well done, 16
social significance of, 16
staff in, 19
starting, 19–20
taking charge in, 15–16
time management in, 16
kitchen shears, 222
knives, 221–22

lactation, 118, 120–21
    alternatives to, 121
    beer and, 120
    nutrient needs in, 120
lacto-ovo vegetarian diet, 115–17
Laetrile (vitamin B-17), 53
lamb, 189
Lappé, Frances Moore, 117
leftovers, 234–41
    beans, 195
    beef, 188
    cookbook indexes and, 236
    freezing, 240
    as lunches, 133, 134
    microwave ovens and, 214
    planning for, 235–38
    sample plans for, 237–38
    as sandwich fillings, 133
    storage of, 239–40
    waste of, 234
legumes, 44
    see also specific legumes
Lexington Market (Baltimore, Md.),
    167
Libby's new products, 175, 253
lighting, dining area, 245–46
lignin, 37–38
linoleic acid, 47
linolenic acid, 47
lipoproteins, 40, 50–51
lunches, 132–40
    beverages in, 134–35
    cost of, 135
    dieter's, 137–40
    in restaurants, 138–40
    salad bars, 139
    sandwiches, 132–34
    school program for, 136

skipping, 93–94
storage of, 134
"zippered" oranges in, 135
lunch meats, 135

magnesium, 78
mannitol, 34
margarine, 48
    butter vs., 179
    diet, 150
Marilyn (crisis eater), 141–42, 144
meat, see protein foods group; specific
    types
"meat" loaf, beans in, 195
men:
    ideal weights for, 83
    muscle weight in, 85
    overweight in, 89
menus:
    66-gram protein, 46
    93-gram protein, 45
    in typical poor diet (table), 73
    see also planning meals and menus
metabolism, 23
    of simple vs. complex
        carbohydrates, 34
    variations in efficiency of, 95
    vitamins and, 52
Metropolitan Life Insurance
    Company, 81, 83
Mexican Meal (contingency plan),
    145
microwave ovens, 213, 214–15
milk, milk products, 176–78
    cooking with, 149
    dried or canned, 177–78
    flavored, 177
    imitation, 176–77
    pasteurized, 176
    vitamin D fortified, 55
millet, 181–82
minerals, 23, 59–71
    analyzing levels of, 66
    deficiencies of, 23, 77–78
    importance of, 59
    purpose of, 23, 77–78
    trace, 65–71
    see also specific minerals
mineral supplements, 64, 71–72

molasses, 32
monounsaturated fats, 48
Mother Hubbard's cupboard, 145–47
mucilages, 37, 38

Naisbitt, John, 79, 252
National Academy of Sciences, 23,
    33, 58
National Cancer Institute, 33, 38,
    106
National Heart, Lung and Blood
    Institute, 49
National Restaurant Association,
    254
New Product News, 253
niacin, 58, 76
nickel, 59
nitrites, 189
nitrogen, 41–42
nouvelle cuisine, 153
NutraSweet, 34
nutrient density, 27
nutrients, 21–28
    in digestion, 23
    dollar-wise foods dense in, 203–4
    energy supplied by, 23
    excessive intake of, 27–28, 74–78
    food labels and, 26–27
    necessary (table), 74–78
    recommended daily allowance of,
        23–26
    see also specific nutrients
nutrition, 21–79
    calories in, *see* calories
    carbohydrates in, 29–40, 74
    component criteria in, 79
    eating habits and, 21–22
    fats in, 46–51, 74
    in lactation, 120
    minerals in, 23, 59–71, 77–78
    in pregnancy, 120
    proteins in, 40–46, 74
    successful, 257–58
    varying food intake in, 21, 28
    vitamin/mineral supplements in,
        64, 71–72
    vitamins in, 23, 51–58, 75–77
    see also specific food groups and topics

office, snacking at, 130, 131
oils, 48–49
    see also fats and oils group
"Okie beans," 195
Onassis, Jacqueline, 245
Orange Fizzle vs. Orange Soda, 166
oranges, "zippers" on, 135
Oriental Stir Fry, 146–47
osteoporosis, 63
outdoor meals, 243
overweight, 80–99
    in aging, 87–88
    body fat measured in, 85–87
    body frame and, 82–83
    career success and, 88–89
    of efficient vs. inefficient energy-
        users, 95
    fitness vs. fatness in, 83–85
    health risk in, 80, 81
    height and weight chart and, 83
    life expectancy and, 81–82
    in men, 89
    prejudices against, 88–89
    source of calories and, 91–93
    total fat cells in, 94
    unhappiness and, 80–81
    in women, 89–90

PABA (para-aminobenzoic acid), 53
pangamic acid (vitamin B-15), 53
paper goods, 244–45
    purchased in bulk, 208–9
Pareto Time Principle, 206
paring knives, 221–22
Pasta del Mar (White and Red),
    146
Pasta Primavera, 145
pastas, 183–84
Pattern I meal plan, 111
    sample meal plan for, 112
    sample menus for, 125
    vegetarian, 113–19, 128
    work sheet for, 260
Pattern II meal plan, 111–13
    sample meal plan for, 114
    sample menus for, 126
    vegetarian, 113–19, 128
    work sheet for, 261

Pattern III meal plan, 113
  lacto-ovo vegetarian diet and, 115–116
  sample meal plan for, 116
  sample menus for, 127
  vegetarian, 113–19, 128
  work sheet for, 262
Pauling, Linus, 56
peanut butter, 133, 196
pectins, 37, 38
peelers, swivel-blade, 221
pellagra, 23
phosphorus, 62–64, 77
  sources of, 63
physical activities, see exercise
pinch tests, 86–87
place mats, 244
planning meals and menus, 100–128
  balanced diet in, 101
  calorie needs in, 101–2
  carbohydrate foods group in, 107–108
  checklist for, 266
  complicated meals in, 123
  crisis eating vs., 141–44
  dairy foods group in, 104
  evolution of, 100
  fats and oils group in, 108, 109
  food-group servings in, 110
  foods selected in, 101, 123–24
  fruit group in, 104–5
  helpers' skills in, 123
  importance of, 100
  improvised ingredients and, 147–148
  in infant feeding, 121–22
  lactation and, 118, 120–21
  leftovers in, 235–36
  lunches, 132–40
  meatless meals in, 113–19, 128
  Pattern I in, 111, 112, 118, 125
  Pattern II in, 111–13, 114, 118, 126
  Pattern III in, 113, 115–16, 118, 127
  patterns in, 101, 110–11
  portion sizes in, 103
  in pregnancy, 118–20
  protein foods group in, 106–7
  purchasing supplies and, 158–59
  snacks, 129–32
  surprise visitors and, 144–48
  vegetable group in, 105
  vegetarian diets in, 115–18, 119, 128
PM/Evening Magazine, 199–200
Point of Purchase Advertising Institute, 207
polysaccharides, storage, 37, 38
polyunsaturated fats, 48
  daily requirement of, 47
  vitamin E and, 56
popcorn, gourmet, 253–54
popcorn poppers, 223
Popsicles, fruit-juice, 130
pork, 188–89
  in commercially prepared products, 190–92
  cooking, 150–51
  cured and smoked, 189
portion sizes, 103
potassium, 59–60, 77
potassium scintillation, body fat measured by, 85
potatoes, 186–87
pots and pans, 211–13
  cleanup of, 229
  gauge of metal in, 211
  type of metal in, 211–12
poultry, 189–90
  in commercially prepared products, 190–92
  cooking, 150–51
  leftover, 237
pregnancy:
  alcohol intake in, 39–40
  artificial sweeteners in, 33
  calcium metabolism in, 63
  calorie needs in, 119
  dieting in, 120
  folate supplements in, 58
  iodine intake in, 70
  iron demands in, 68
  menu planning in, 118–20
  nutrient needs in, 120
  Pattern II meal plan in, 112
  weight gain in, 119–20

preparing food, 223–29
　in advance, 223–25, 227
　organization in, 225–27, 228
　simple vs. complex recipes in, 227
　timing in, 225–26
presentation of food, 241–50
　arrangement on plate in, 247
　centerpieces in, 245
　color schemes in, 244
　effect of, 241–42
　lighting in, 245–46
　location of, 243
　names chosen for, 249–50
　place mats in, 244
　shapes of food cut in, 247
　table settings in, 242
　trends as inspiration for, 251–58
　variety of colors in, 246–47
　variety of textures in, 248
preservatives, food, 201–2
pressure cookers, 216–17
prime grade meats, 188
"Princess Pudding," 236
processed foods, 61–62
produce, see canned produce; fruits;
　vegetables
protein foods group, 106–7, 264
　commercially prepared products in,
　　190–92
　purchasing supplies from, 187–96
proteins, 40–46
　affluence and intake of, 40–41
　animal, 42–43, 44
　in beans, 195
　calcium intake and, 63
　chemical composition of, 41
　complementary, 43, 117
　complete, 42
　deficient intake of, 42, 74
　excessive intake of, 42, 44–46, 74
　fat intake and, 42, 44, 45, 107
　importance of, 41
　incomplete, 43
　metabolism of, 41–42
　plant food sources of, 42–44
　in vegetarian diets, 43, 44, 116–17
provitamins, 54, 55
purchasing supplies, 154–204
　advertisements and, 159

beans, 194–95
beef, 187–88
best nutritional buys in, 203–4
breads, 182–83
in bulk, 160, 167, 208–9
butter, 179
cakes and cookies, 187
canned produce, 170–75
cereals, 185
cheese, 179–80, 181
commercially prepared meat
　products, 190–92
continuous inventories in, 157–58
convenience foods, 197–201
crackers, 184
delivery of, 161
dry goods, 208–9
eggs, 192–93
egg substitutes, 193–94
fabricated foods, 201–3
fake foods, 196–97
fish, 192
fresh produce, 166–70
frozen produce, 170–75
impulsiveness in, 159
juices, 164–65
lamb, 189
margarine, 179
menu plan and, 158–59
milk products, 176–78
nonperishable staples, 158
ongoing list for, 157
pastas, 183–84
peanut butter, 196
plan, 157
pork, 188–89
potatoes, 186–87
poultry, 189–90
prices compared in, 154
quality grades vs. use considered
　in, 155
rice, 185–86
seasonal availability and, 171–73
shopping list for, 266–67
soft drinks, 165–66
in specialty stores, 160
stores in, 159–61
time management in, 207–9
tofu, 180

tortillas, 185
"twofer" sales and, 163
unit pricing in, 162–63
variety of choices in, 163–64
in warehouse stores, 160
weekly food costs in, 155–57
whole grain foods, 181–82
yogurt, 178
pyridoxine (vitamin B-6), 58, 76

quality grading systems:
of beef, 187–88
of canned and frozen produce, 170–171
of eggs, 192–93
of fresh produce, 166–67
of pork, 188
of poultry, 189–90

radioactive tracer dyes, body fat measured by, 85
Recipes for a Small Planet (Lappé), 117
Recommended Daily Allowances (RDA), 23–26
food labels and, 26–27
periodic revision of, 257
restaurant meals:
chef's time management in, 227–229
"dieter's plates" in, 138
dieting and, 137–40
dinners, 140
fast food, 138
low-calorie selections in, 254
nouvelle cuisine in, 153
salad bars in, 139
substitutions in, 139–40
wine in, 140
riboflavin (vitamin B-2), 58, 76
rice, 185–86
brown, 186
rickets, 23
rutin, 53

saccharin, 33
salad bars, 139, 254
salad dressings, 139
low-fat, 150
salad dryers, 220–21

Salazar, Alberto, 85
salt, 61–62
in baby foods, 122
in canned and frozen produce, 174–175
in carrots, 175
in cheese, 180
in cooking, 151–52
in fabricated foods, 201
iodized, 69–70
in meats, 189
salts, mineral, 59
sandwiches, 132–34
dieter's, 137
peanut butter, 196
saturated fats, 48, 51
sauces, low-fat, 149
ready-made, 175
served on side, 247–48
scalloped knives, 222
school lunch programs, 136
selenium, 66–67, 78
serrated blade knives, 222
sex hormones, 49
shopping lists, 207, 208, 266–67
simple carbohydrates, see sugar
skillets, cast iron, 212
skillets, electric, 215
skinfold calipers, 86–87
slow cookers, 215, 216
smokers, vitamin C and, 57
snacking, 129–32
calories hidden in, 131–32
cleanup after, 230
dieting and, 111, 131
distractions avoided in, 130
fruits vs. treats in, 104–5, 109, 170
hurried, 129–30
"midmorning Blahs" and, 31–32
nutrition as goal in, 131
scheduling, 130
sodium, 59–62
sources of, 61–62
in water regulation, 59–61
see also salt
soft drinks, 30, 165
alternatives to, 166
fructose in, 33
trends in, 253

sonograms, body fat measured by, 85
sorbitol, 34
SOS eating, 106
Southwestern Bread Pie, 147
spices, 152
staples, 164–96
    beans, 194–95
    beef, 187–88
    breads, 182–83
    butter or margarine, 179
    canned produce, 170–75
    cereals, 185
    cheese, 179–80, 181
    convenience foods, 197–201
    crackers, 184
    eggs, 192–93
    fabricated foods, 201–3
    fish, 192
    fresh produce, 166–70
    frozen produce, 170–75
    juices, 164
    lamb, 189
    milk products, 176–78
    orange juice, 164–65
    pastas, 183–84
    peanut butter, 196
    pork, 188–89
    potatoes, 186–87
    poultry, 189–90
    rice, 185–86
    soft drinks, 165–66
    tofu, 180
    tortillas, 185
    treats, 187
    whole grain foods, 181–82
    yogurt, 178
starch foods, 29, 34–37
    blood sugar level and, 34–35
    diets high in, 36–37
    diets low in, 35–36
    fats served with, 35–36
    metabolism of, 34
    nutrients in, 35
    thiamine in, 57
stir-frying, 216
"stock box," 240
storage:
    containers for, 239–40
    of fish, 192

    of lettuce, 220–21, 224
    of lunches, 134
    in stores, 161
stores, 159–63
    appearance of, 160
    congested periods in, 208
    convenience, 161–62
    delicatessens, 161–62
    kitchen supply, 210
    price variations among, 159–60
    sanitation in, 161
    services offered by, 160–61
    specialty, 160
    "twofer" sales in, 163
    unit pricing in, 162–63
    see also suppliers
"strippers," 221
successful nutrition, 257–58
sugar, 29–34
    abusive intake of, 31
    in baby foods, 122
    blood sugar and, 92–93
    brown, 32
    in canned and frozen produce, 174
    in cereals, 185
    in cooking and baking, 152–53
    in fabricated foods, 201
    on food labels, 30–31
    in juices, 165
    sources of, 29–30
    substitutes for, 33–34
    tooth decay and, 31
sunlight, vitamin D production and,
    55
suppliers:
    farmers' markets, 167
    local growers, 166–67
    produce terminals, 167
    see also stores

table settings, 242–46
    centerpieces, 245
    colors in, 244
    coverings, 243–44
    lighting, 245–46
    place mats, 244
telephone answering machines, 207
Terminal Market (San Francisco,
    Calif.), 167

thermos containers, 134–35
thiamine (vitamin B-1), 57, 76
time management, 16, 205–33
  advance preparation in, 223–25, 227
  assistance in, 209, 231–33
  in cleanup chores, 229–33
  delegating responsibility in, 209, 231–33, 267–70
  distractions in, 207
  efficient techniques in, 207
  kitchen equipment in, 210–23
  leftovers in, 236
  meal plan in, 207
  in organizing meal preparation, 225–29
  plan needed in, 205–7
  routine tasks in, 206–7
  in shopping, 207–9
  shopping list in, 207, 208, 266–67
T-lymphocytes, 65
toaster-ovens, 213–14
toasters, 213
"toddler" foods, 122
tofu, 103, 151, 180–81
  in infant feeding, 121
Tofutti, 181
tooth decay, 31
tortillas, 185
tray tables, 243
treats group, 108–9, 266
  fabricated foods, 201–3
  fruits vs., 104–5, 109, 170
  leftover, 236
  purchasing, 187
trends, 251–58
  celebrity endorsements of, 256
  competitiveness in, 255–56
  "exotic," 254
  family changes and, 251–52
  in fast foods, 254–55
  gourmet, 253–54
  "health," 253
  low-calorie, 253
  new products in, 79, 253
  no-caffeine, 253
  social setting of, 252, 255–56
  spotting, 255
trichinosis, 188–89

tuna recipes (contingency plan), 146
TV dinners, 198–99
Twinkies, 202
"twofer" sales, 163

unsaturated fats, 48
USRDA, 26–27

vegan diet, 115, 117–18
  sample meal plan for, 119
  sample menus for, 128
vegetable group, 105–6, 264
  purchasing staples from, 164–75
vegetables:
  appearance of, 168
  bulk purchases of, 167
  canned, 170–75
  "exotic," 254
  fatty acids in, 48
  frozen, 170–75
  grading of, 167–68
  hints for selection of, 168
  leftover, 237
  locally grown, 166–67
  peelings, 221
  in produce terminals, 167
  with sauce or gravy, 175
  seasonal availability of, 171–73
  storage of, 168
vegetarians, 42, 115–18
  animal protein eschewed by, 113–115
  calcium intake of, 117
  iron intake of, 117
  lacto-ovo, 115–17
  meal plans for, 113–19, 128
  protein sources for, 43, 44, 116–17
  vegans, 115, 117–18, 119, 128
  vitamin B-12 and, 58
vinegars, 163
vitamin A, 47, 54, 75
vitamin B-1 (thiamine), 57, 76
vitamin B-2 (riboflavin), 58, 76
vitamin B-6 (pyridoxine), 58, 76
vitamin B-12 (cobalamin), 58, 77
vitamin C (ascorbic acid), 56–57, 76
  iron absorption and, 69
Vitamin C and the Common Cold (Pauling), 56

vitamin D, 47, 54–55, 75
  cholesterol and, 49
vitamin deficiency syndromes, 52, 75–
    77
vitamin E, 47, 55–56, 75
  selenium and, 66
vitamin K, 47, 56, 75
vitamins, 51–58
  deficiencies of, 23, 52–53, 75–77
  excessive intake of, 53, 75–77
  fat-soluble, 47, 53, 54–56, 75
  importance of, 51–52
  "nonvitamins," 53
  purpose of, 23
  research on, 53
  toxic levels of, 53, 54
  water-soluble, 53
  see also specific vitamins
vitamin supplements, 71–72

waffle irons, 223
Waitz, Grete, 85
water, fluoridated, 70–71
weight, 80–99
  body frame and, 82–83
  changes in ideals of, 89–90
  fitness and, 83–85
  ideal, 28, 81–84
  ideal, for adults, 83
  ideal, for children, 84
  life expectancy and, 81–82

  of men, 89
  percentage of, as fat, 85–87
  physical activity and, 95–99
  sugar substitutes and, 33–34
  of women, 89–90
Wendy's International, 253–54
wheat berries, 181–82
whole grain foods, 181–82
Wisconsin, Medical College of, 83,
    84
woks, electric, 215–16
Woman's Day, 157
women:
  aging in, 87–88
  ideal weights for, 83
  iron deficiency in, 67–68
  lactating, see lactation
  muscle weight in, 85
  overweight in, 89–90
  pregnant, see pregnancy

X-rays, body fat measured by, 85
xylitol, 34

Yankelovich Skelly and White, 251
yogurt:
  homemade, 178
  purchasing, 178
  sour cream replaced by, 149

zinc, 65–66, 77
  toxic levels of, 66